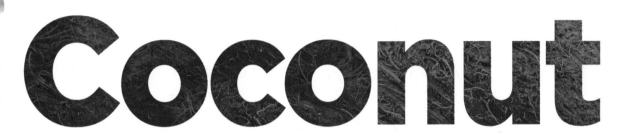

# Coconut

*To my guys: Leif Christian Pedersen,*
*Anders Gyldenvalde Pedersen, Axel SuneLund Pedersen,*
*and Richard Joseph Demler. I adore you.*

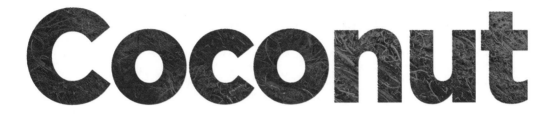

# Coconut

## The Complete Guide to the
## World's Most Versatile Superfood

**STEPHANIE PEDERSEN**

STERLING
New York

STERLING
New York

An Imprint of Sterling Publishing
1166 Avenue of the Americas
New York, NY 10036

Text © 2015 by Stephanie Pedersen

Photo Credits: Cover and interior color photography by Bill Milne, © Sterling Publishing; Additional interior credits: Corbis Images: © Radius Images 124; iStockPhoto: © AK2 156, © Aluxum 146, © Amriphoto 173, © Bonchan 159, © Cislander xii, © Cjrfoto 135, © Creativeye99 137, © Luigi DiMaggio 85, © DNY59 102, © Duckycards 153, © Floortje 3, © Christine Glade 145, © Hid_de 149, © Hudiemm 61, © iSailorr 97, © Robyn Mac 82, © Matejay 60 © Ntstudio 55, © Ockra 73, © john shepherd 111, © Songsak Paname xi, © Lauri Patterson 110, © Joanna Pecha 65, © Pesky Monkey 48, © Picture Partners 105, 160, © Princess Lisa, 56, © Savany, 70, © sitriel 25, © Julia Sudnitskaya 117, © szefei 57, © softservegirl 143, © Subjug, 69, © Syolacan, 99, © taseffski 47, © Alasdair Thomson 35, © Tiverylucky 4, © Watcha 129; Shutterstock: © DeeaF109, © Kitty 29

Interior Design by Philip Buchanan

ISBN 978-1-4549-1340-5

Distributed in Canada by Sterling Publishing
℅ Canadian Manda Group, 664 Annette Street
Toronto, Ontario, Canada M6S 2C8
Distributed in the United Kingdom by GMC Distribution Services
Castle Place, 166 High Street, Lewes, East Sussex, England BN7 1XU
Distributed in Australia by Capricorn Link (Australia) Pty. Ltd.
P.O. Box 704, Windsor, NSW 2756, Australia

For information about custom editions, special sales, and premium and corporate purchases, please contact Sterling Special Sales at 800-805-5489 or specialsales@sterlingpublishing.com.

Manufactured in Canada

2 4 6 8 10 9 7 5 3 1

www.sterlingpublishing.com

# CONTENTS

# INTRODUCTION

As a young girl I lived in Australia, a place where coconuts are everywhere, even though they are not native to Australia and are not grown commercially there. In fact, they grow only sparsely along Oz's northern coast . . . and yet, Australians eat coconuts in large quantities. Yes, Aussies are coconut lovers. Go Down Under and you'll find the famous Anzac biscuits, coconut shortbread, lamingtons (small squares of cake dipped in chocolate and coated with coconut), coconut sponge, baked coconut pudding, Cherry Ripe chocolate bars (with cherries and coconut), and my favorite, Europe Apricot & Coconut bars, as well as other coconut-heavy sweets.

For me, as I was growing up, coconut was a delectable, sweet food that I associated with good times and treats. I didn't used to think of it as an ingredient that could be eaten in a wide range of dishes. And I certainly didn't grow up with the idea that coconut was good for you.

I was a child in the 1970s and '80s, a time of margarine, aspartame, and no-fat diets. Most people in Australia, the United States, and Europe (the cultures my family and I lived in) had never heard of coconut water, and we certainly didn't cook with coconut oil. The only dried coconut we ever saw was coated with sweetener and packaged in a blue plastic bag. And the idea of cooking with flour that wasn't made from wheat seemed unthinkable. In other words, it was a different time. In fact, I didn't see an actual, mature coconut until I was in my late teens, when my dad brought one home after winning it as a gag gift at work. It was only when I became an adult, and began regularly traveling to the West Indies, that I laid eyes upon a green coconut for the first time.

I don't think my coconut experience—or lack thereof—was uncommon.

My mother got her nutrition information from women's magazines, which told her that saturated fats were the enemy—so out went red meat and butter. Tropical oils were shunned, too; nutrition experts from that time told us coconut oil was the most dangerous fat possible. Thus, entire generations grew up without coconut oil and ate foods made with *more acceptable* hydrogenated vegetable shortening and margarine instead.

The first time I was exposed to thinking about alternative fats was in my twenties, when I was working in New York City as a kitchen assistant at the Natural Gourmet Institute, the renowned whole foods cooking school, where revolutionary natural food chefs such as Peter Brearley, Myra Kornfeld Elliott Prag, and Diane Carlson taught. My job was twofold: to help cooking instructors get ready for class by prepping ingredients, and to ensure that their classes ran smoothly by performing the backstage work (everything from fetching ingredients for the instructor to washing dishes).

One particular day, during an introductory lesson on whole food ingredients, instructor Diane Carlson mentioned that studies were beginning to show that coconut oil and other coconut products had powerful healing properties and were not harmful to the heart, as many people believed at the time. She passed around a few handouts on heart disease rates in Southeast Asian and West Indian countries, where coconut oil, coconut milk, and coconut meat were consumed in large quantities, as opposed to Canada and the United States, where consumption of hydrogenated vegetable shortening and margarine were the norm. The studies showed that Southeast Asian and West Indian heart disease rates were low compared to those of the Western world.

This was new.

Wanting to get every drop of wisdom we could get on coconut oil, we kitchen assistants leapt into action: One of us took frantic notes while the rest of us continued chopping, stirring, and washing dishes.

After the class was over and we'd cleaned the kitchen, we raced to a copy shop to photocopy our notes. We had a quest: find out everything we could about coconut oil.

We searched the cooking school's library shelves and pored over back issues of every healing and natural food magazine we could find. A few of us hit the public library. These were the early days of the Internet, so hopping online, as all of us did, and searching for "Coconut Oil," led us straight to a bunch of alternative health websites that were so zealous, we couldn't be sure where enthusiasm wore off and accuracy began.

What I was looking for was reassurance—proof, even—that I was not going to doom myself to a life of heart disease by regularly consuming coconut. Finally, I felt that I'd read enough; I was convinced that the product was not health threatening, and I was ready to take the plunge. Unfortunately, finding coconut oil proved to be more challenging than unearthing reliable research.

One of my friends brought back an unmarked jar of coconut oil from a trip to Barbados. She had no idea if it was cold-pressed or if the coconut that was used to make the oil was organic, but at last we had some! We split the oil among the three of us and took it home.

The first thing I did with the coconut oil was make a vegetable curry, which I finished off with a cup of coconut milk. I figured if coconut oil was good for me, coconut milk must be, too! I had been using extra-virgin olive oil for everything prior to this; the coconut oil made the dish taste so much more authentic. It was absolutely delicious.

I used the oil every day, until it ran out, to bake, roast veggies, and make salad dressings. I even used it to make popcorn and rubbed it into my hair and skin, like many of my friends from "coconut countries" did. I had found a new love. I adored the well-rounded, nutty, buttery flavor that coconut oil brought to everything I cooked, and was in awe of all the protein, fiber, calcium, iron, magnesium, manganese, potassium, zinc, vitamin C, B-complex vitamins, phytonutrients, fatty acids, amino acids, electrolytes, and antimicrobial elements this nourishing food contains.

In those early days at the Natural Gourmet Institute, my experimentation with coconut showed me that it is indeed a powerful and delicious everyday ingredient. I began by using a range of coconut products, including coconut milk, dried coconut, and fresh green and mature brown coconuts. I tried coconut water for the first time, and started to make my own coconut milk and dry my own shredded coconut. Later, when the gluten-free movement started and coconut flour became available, I jumped at the chance to play with another coconut ingredient. And when I discovered coconut nectar and coconut sugar, I pulled out my muffin tins and began to experiment. But experimentation didn't stop there; when I stumbled upon coconut vinegar and coconut aminos, out came the blender, allowing me to whip up a flurry of marinades, sauces, and dressings.

Today I enjoy coconut, in one form or another, at almost every meal. I use coconut water to make ice cubes and rely on coconut milk to replace dairy in just about every single recipe I make. I have been known to sneak coconut oil into my dog's food to treat his itchy skin, and have even used coconut butter, whipped with coconut nectar, to make an impromptu frosting for cupcakes. Even as I write this introduction, I have one hand on my keyboard and the other in a bowl of popcorn popped in coconut oil.

Along the way, I've learned a few wonderful things firsthand:

• Coconut oil, coconut meat, coconut flour, and coconut milk have reduced my cravings for sweets, probably by improving insulin secretion and utilization of blood glucose. The healthy fat in coconut has been shown to slow elevations in blood sugar and reduce hypoglycemic cravings.

- Coconut nectar and coconut sugar boast a low glycemic index, which leaves my kids happy, without the "sugar hyperactivity" they exhibit directly after eating anything made with cane sugar. Plus, there is no grouchy "post-sugar crash" with coconut sweeteners. For me, this alone makes coconut a miracle ingredient.

- Coconut improves immune system function. Before I added coconut to my oldest son's diet, he was getting sick from a virus almost every month. After adding two or three servings of coconut oil, coconut flour, and coconut milk to his everyday diet, he started catching only one or two colds a year, thanks to the antioxidant content of coconut.

- The antioxidant effects of coconut can help protect your skin from cellular damage from ultraviolet light, while the medium chain fatty acids in coconut help strengthen connective tissue—the results of which can be beautiful-looking skin.

- A naturopath friend mentioned that the medium chain fatty acids in coconut could help increase my metabolism and improve thyroid function while strengthening my sluggish adrenal gland function. A year after incorporating tablespoons of coconut oil into my diet each day, plus coconut water, coconut milk, and coconut flour most days, my adrenal gland function returned to normal.

- The electrolytes in coconut water help hydrate my husband on his runs in a more natural way than chemical-heavy sports drinks.

- Coconut flour and coconut meat contain generous amounts of fiber, which fills the tummy, leaving me so satisfied I'm not interested in after-meal snacking.

Although I have not suffered from a heart condition, high cholesterol, cancer, or a neurological disease, my research has uncovered several studies that suggest that coconut's many nutrients help prevent and heal these conditions. One—the 2003 study performed by a team out of the School of Dietetics and Human Nutrition, McGill University in Quebec—found that overweight women who consumed a diet rich in medium chain fatty acids (the primary ingredient in coconut oil) enjoyed lowered cholesterol levels than those who received the majority of their fat from beef. (I come from a family of beef-eaters, so this study was of great interest to me!) A team at the same research site, after reviewing human and animal studies on coconut oil, and the medium chain fatty acids it contains, concluded that fats, such as coconut oil, that are rich in medium chain fatty acids may result in faster satiety and facilitate weight control when included in the diet as a replacement for fats containing long chain fatty acids—the fatty acids in animal and hydrogenated fats. Coconut is indeed a "superfood," and a popular one at that. Check out any raw food, Paleo, or gluten-free blog; vegan restaurant; vegetarian magazine; or alternative health website, and you'll find anecdotal proof that coconut is the darling of the health set.

I have my own unofficial proof that coconut is one of the health world's most popular power foods: When I began writing *Coconut*, I quizzed my nutritionist and natural health friends on the foods they eat every single day (at least once, if not two or three times a day) to stay healthy. Coconut was the only food that all 226 of them ate daily in some form or another. Furthermore, each September I host the Superfood Superheroes Summit, an online education event, during which I spend a week interviewing superfood authors and other experts. Last year when I asked each health pro to share a recipe, the only superfood ingredient that every single expert's recipe included was coconut. That's pretty telling, right?

No matter how you crack it, coconut tastes amazing, is easy to find, and is wonderful for use in a staggering array of delicious recipes, from smoothies and juices to main dishes and little dishes, to baked goods and desserts—complete with the lovely bonus of health benefits that will keep you and your family as healthy and vibrant as possible. Taste, versatility, and health benefits—how many ingredients do you know that offer as many desirable qualities?

Throughout this book, you'll find plenty of tips on choosing, using, and storing your precious coconut ingredients, as well as tricks to help you make your own coconut staples. (Anyone want to know how to make Coconut Cream Dessert Topping or homemade coconut milk?) I've tried to keep the recipes as healthy as possible, which in my world means whole food ingredients, a minimum of dairy and wheat, and lots of plant food. If applicable, substitutions and alternative options are noted within the recipe, along with details about any unusual steps or storage advice.

It's a great time for coconut, and if you are ready to dive in and experience the wonders of coconut yourself, it's all here.

With love and coconut bliss to all of you,
Stephanie Pedersen, MS, CHHC, AADP
Holistic Nutritionist

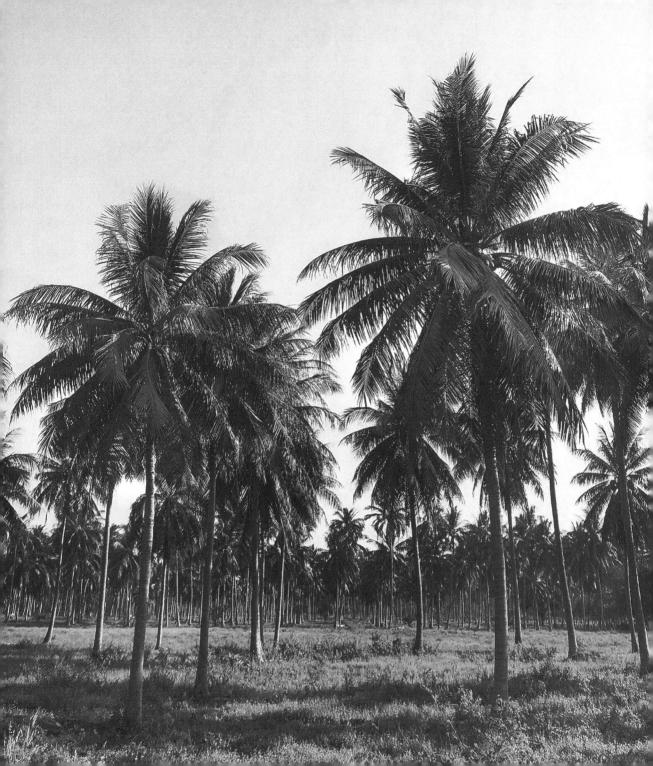

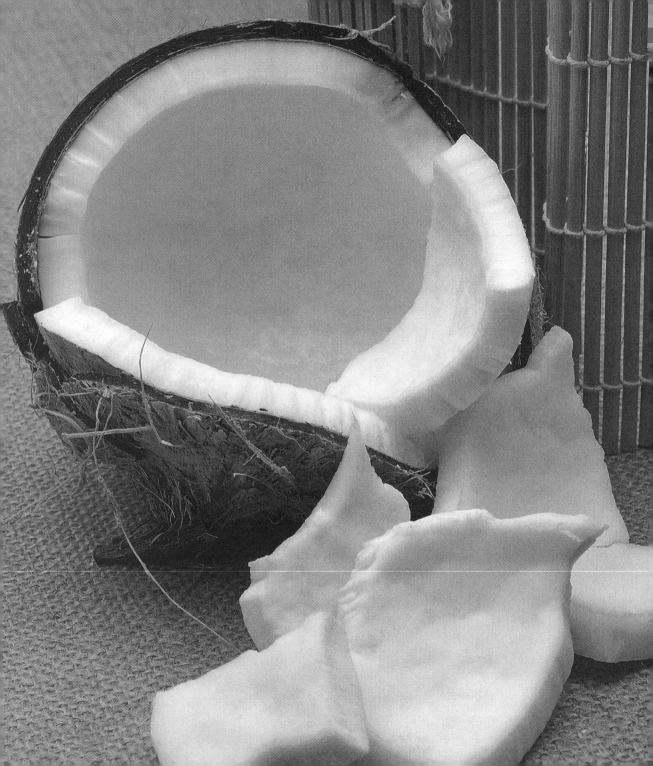

# CHAPTER 1

# GETTING FRIENDLY WITH COCONUT

Hello coconut lovers! I am so excited to share one of my favorite superfoods with you, as well as welcome all of you healthy folks who have heard that coconut is a great way to boost your health and make sure your family gets the nutrition they need to be their best. And friendly greetings to those of you who are not coconut fans, but are here because you love someone who loves coconut, or because your doctor or nutritionist told you that you need to eat more coconut.

Coconut comes in many different forms, including coconut water, fresh coconut meat, dried coconut meat, coconut oil, coconut milk, coconut flour, coconut sweeteners, coconut vinegar, and more. I hope you'll try them all. You may be like me and love every single one of these, or you may prize one ingredient above the rest. While coconut flour has different benefits than coconut water, which in turn, has a different nutrient profile than coconut oil, all coconut foods are worthy additions to your daily diet.

That's what I tell my clients: Try for at least one coconut product every day. Each coconut product has a different host of nutrients. If you can enjoy at least one coconut product every day, you'll end each week in a powerful, healthful place.

### COCONUT'S ANCIENT ORIGINS

One of the earliest descriptions of the coconut palm was written in about 545 CE, in *Topographia Christiana*, a work by Cosmas, who made several trips to India and was famous for his maps of the world.

Still, the origins of the coconut remain a mystery: Scientists have used art, fossils, genetics, and travel records to figure out where the coconut first appeared.

Odoardo Beccari, a renowned palm specialist during the late 1800s and early 1900s, suggested that the coconut is of Southeast Pacific origin. Strengthening his argument is the fact that there are more varieties of coconut palms in the Eastern Hemisphere than in the Americas. However, no conclusive evidence exists, so for now, we'll have to be content with coconut's great taste, versatility, and health benefits.

As you've probably already noticed, coconut is absolutely everywhere! Coconut oil, which was, at one time, relegated to skin care, has been a hot food for decades now, as more and more families of autistic children and Alzheimer's patients have touted its ability to help normalize brain and nervous system function. At the same time, cardiologists and others who are concerned with heart health have found coconut to be effective in helping heal cardiovascular disorders, while IBS (irritable bowel syndrome) sufferers and individuals with other digestive disorders have found coconut oil to be helpful in healing their damaged large intestine.

Coconut water, the fastest-growing beverage in the world, first appeared in US supermarkets in 2004. The popularity of this refreshing drink is borne out by these statistics from the data resource company Euromonitor: Sales of the highest-selling brands in the United States—Vita Coco, ZICO, and O.N.E., which control the vast majority of the American coconut water market—have skyrocketed by nearly 600 percent since 2009, and 2,759 percent since 2007.

Coconut milk is now available in convenient cartons right next to dairy milk, and has become a favorite of vegans and others who "don't do" dairy. In the United Kingdom, sales of nondairy alternatives (including coconut milk) have risen by 40 percent in the last three years—with similar numbers in the United States. Coconut flour, too, has grown in popularity, thanks to the rising number of gluten-free consumers and individuals who follow the Paleo diet, which eschews grains and grain-based flours in favor of high-fiber, high-protein, low-carbohydrate whole foods that nourish the body without causing bloat and inflammation.

The high reputation of low glycemic coconut sugar and coconut nectar, as alternatives to other sugars, has arrived hot on the heels of data released by the American Diabetes Association that shows nearly twenty-six million children and adults in the United States have diabetes and seventy-nine million Americans have prediabetes. These individuals must find ways to eat that don't cause dangerous fluctuations in their blood sugar—their lives literally depend upon it.

If you've been motivated to find products like apple cider vinegar—with its alkalizing, anti-inflammatory powers—to help you feel energetic and craving-free, you'll soon discover that coconut vinegar has the same superpowers. And, as more people become aware of the dangers of overusing soy, coconut aminos has become the go-to replacement for soy sauce and Bragg Liquid Aminos.

Last, there are coconut specialty products like coconut cream and coconut butter—even actual fresh young coconuts and mature coconuts—which add nutrient-dense luxury to even the most pious diet.

No matter which coconut product you try, one of the best, foolproof ways to be sure you and your loved ones enjoy a daily serving of coconut is to start with the best-quality coconut products you can find. The first step in doing that is to "buy smart."

Whether you are shopping for coconut milk or coconut vinegar, the fewer ingredients on the label the better. Like many other natural products, coconut milk, coconut flour, coconut water, and myriad other coconut products are often meddled with and altered with the addition of water, sweeteners, unnecessary flavorings, chemical preservatives, emulsifiers, stabilizers, anticaking agents, colorants, and more. None of these additives are necessary. Look for pure products in their most natural state and you will always do well.

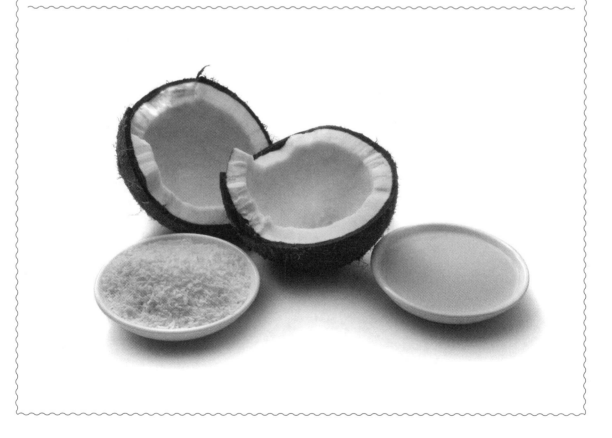

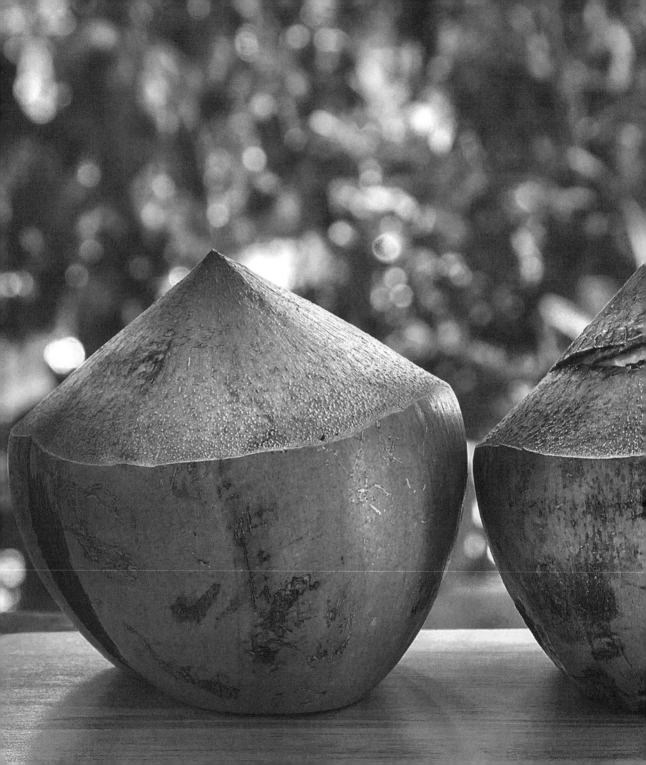

# CHAPTER 2

# COCONUT: THE EVERYDAY POWERHOUSE

I call coconut an "everyday food" because it comes in so many forms and offers such a wide range of nutrients, so it's easy—and smart—for you to enjoy daily. In my household, we eat coconut in one form or another at just about every meal and snack. This gives us a generous helping of the nutrients we need to stay healthy and keeps the adults in the household looking and feeling young, vibrant, and slim, while keeping all of our immune, cardiovascular, and nervous systems strong and efficient.

Fortunately, coconut comes in oils, sweeteners, sauces, flours, and more, making it a cinch to add coconut to our diet. Coconut is also easy to use and lends itself effortlessly to everything from popcorn to salad dressings to smoothies to dinner entrées.

This chapter is dedicated to giving you an idea of the wide range of coconut products that are available, and featured in the recipe section of the book. Here, you'll learn more about the nutritional profile and health benefits of each product, where it comes from, and how it's produced. I'll also suggest tips and tricks for using each ingredient successfully. Enjoy!

## GREEN COCONUT

Up until recently, young, green coconuts were a rarity in the non-coconut-growing world. It was the brown, mature fruit that most of us associated with the word "coconut." Thanks to the raw food and Paleo movements, green coconuts are a common sight in juice joints, health food stores, and supermarkets everywhere. Green coconuts are large and heavy and can be eaten raw: Just hack away the green coating, split it open, drain off the water (don't throw it away, though!), and scoop out the young, gelatinous fruit. Young coconut flesh is slightly sweet and refreshing with a subtle richness, and best of all, it offers a wide range of nutrients.

# GREEN COCONUT: NUTRITION PROFILE PER SERVING (1 CUP)

**CALORIES:** 283

**FIBER:** A serving of fresh coconut provides 7.2 g of fiber, helping promote digestive health and helping you feel full so you eat less. Fiber has been found to lower the risk of certain cancers, such as colorectal cancer and other gastrointestinal cancers.

**PROTEIN:** At 2.66 g of coconut per serving, green coconut has a respectable amount of protein, the macronutrient responsible for helping your body build and repair itself.

**MEDIUM CHAIN FATTY ACIDS:** Like other coconut products, young coconut flesh contains medium chain fatty acids. MCFAs, as these are also known, have shown promise in reducing abdominal obesity and diminishing fat storage.

**LAURIC ACID:** Coconut flesh is also rich in lauric acid, which is known for its bacteria- and virus-killing properties. Lauric acid is also found in breast milk, helping boost newborns' immunity and protecting them against infections.

**POTASSIUM:** This mineral is crucial to body functions. One cup of green coconut flesh provides 285 mg of the recommended dietary allowance of about 4,700 mg.

## RDAS, USDA, AND YOU

In the United States, you often read about RDAs—recommended dietary allowances. Most nutrients are assigned an RDA by the United States Department of Agriculture (USDA). This assigned number represents the ideal average daily intake of the nutrient. You'll find this number referred to as "RDA," "recommended dietary allowance," or "daily requirement." The three terms are used interchangeably throughout this book.

**PHOSPHORUS:** Phosphorus is a mineral that makes up 1 percent of the body's total weight, and it is present in every cell of the body—particularly in bones and teeth. Adults need about 700 mg a day. A serving of young coconut provides 90 mg.

**CALCIUM:** In addition to its well-known role as bone-and-teeth-builder, calcium helps the body's muscles move and enables nerves to carry messages between the brain and other parts of the body. According to the USDA, an adult should get around 1,000 mg per day. Young coconut provides 11 mg per serving.

**MAGNESIUM:** Magnesium is needed for more than three hundred biochemical reactions in the body. It helps maintain normal nerve and muscle function, supports a healthy immune system, keeps the heartbeat steady,

# NUTRIENTS: HOW MUCH DO YOU NEED?

Name a nutrient—any nutrient—and chances are good that different people, of different ages and life stages, and of different genders, need different amounts of it. This is why the United States Department of Agriculture has created nutritional guidelines for most nutrients in the form of RDA (recommended dietary allowance) or AI (adequate intake). Here is a list of nutrients found in coconut products, along with the USDA's intake suggestions. Note: The USDA breaks down recommended dietary allowances into very narrow groups, as well as offering suggestions for larger, more general groups, some of which we share with you here.

**FIBER**
men, over the age of 18: **38 g**
women, over the age of 18: **25 g**
pregnant women: **28 mg**

**PROTEIN**
men, over the age of 18: **56 g**
women, over the age of 18: **26 g**
pregnant women: **71 g**

**VITAMIN A**
men, over the age of 18: **900 IUs**
women, over the age of 18: **700 IUs**
pregnant women: **770 IUs**

**VITAMIN B6**
men, over the age of 18: **1.3 mg**
women, over the age of 18: **1.3 mg**
pregnant women: **1.9 mg**

**VITAMIN C**
men, over the age of 18: **90 mg**
women, over the age of 18: **75 mg**
pregnant women: **85 mg**

**VITAMIN E**
men, over the age of 18: **15 mg**
women, over the age of 18: **15 mg**
pregnant women: **15 mg**

**VITAMIN K**
men, over the age of 18: **120 g**
women, over the age of 18: **90 g**
pregnant women: **90 g**

**FOLATE**
men, over the age of 18: **400 g**
women, over the age of 18: **400 g**
pregnant women: **600 g**

**THIAMINE**
men, over the age of 18: **1.2 mg**
women, over the age of 18: **1.1 mg**
pregnant women: **1.4 mg**

**RIBOFLAVIN**
men, over the age of 18: **1.3 mg**
women, over the age of 18: **1.1 mg**
pregnant women: **1.4 mg**

**NIACIN**
men, over the age of 18: **16 mg**
women, over the age of 18: **14 mg**
pregnant women: **18 mg**

**CALCIUM**
men, over the age of 18: **1,000 mg**
women, over the age of 18: **1,000 mg**
pregnant women: **1,000 mg**

**IRON**
men, over the age of 18: **8 mg**
women, over the age of 18: **18 mg**
pregnant women: **27 mg**

**MAGNESIUM**
men, over the age of 18: **400 mg**
women, over the age of 18: **310 mg**
pregnant women: **350 mg**

**PHOSPHORUS**
men, over the age of 18: **700 mg**
women, over the age of 18: **700 mg**
pregnant women: **700 mg**

**POTASSIUM**
men, over the age of 18: **4.7 g**
women, over the age of 18: **4.7 g**
pregnant women: **4.7 g**

**ZINC**
men, over the age of 18: **11 mg**
women, over the age of 18: **8 mg**
pregnant women: **11 mg**

**SELENIUM**
men, over the age of 18: **55 mcg**
women, over the age of 18: **55 mcg**
pregnant women: **60 mcg**

and helps bones remain strong. Adult women should get around 310 mg of magnesium daily (men should get 400 mg); one serving of young coconut flesh will supply 6 percent of the RDA for this important mineral.

IRON: In addition to its role in red blood cell production, iron is necessary for growth, development, normal cellular functioning, and synthesis of some hormones and connective tissue. Young coconut provides 1.94 mg of the USDA recommended dietary allowance of 8 mg per day for men and 18 mg for women.

MANGANESE: Manganese is an essential nutrient involved in many chemical interactions in the body, including processing cholesterol, carbohydrates, and protein. It may also be involved in bone formation. While no recommended dietary allowance of manganese has been established by the USDA, or any other organization, 1 to 2 mg is considered an adequate daily dosage. Young coconut contains 1.2 mg of manganese per serving.

ZINC: Young coconut provides 0.88 mg of zinc per serving; the recommended dietary allowance is 8 mg for women and 11 mg for men. Zinc plays a role in immune function, protein synthesis, wound healing, DNA synthesis, and cell division.

COPPER: Low copper intake has been associated with high cholesterol and cardiovascular disease in some individuals. While the USDA has not yet determined a daily recommended dietary allowance, it considers 2 mg an adequate daily goal for adults. Young coconut provides 0.348 mg per serving.

SELENIUM: This trace element is necessary for several critical body functions, including reproduction, thyroid hormone metabolism, DNA synthesis, and protection from oxidative damage and infection. The USDA suggests that adults consume 55 mcg daily. Young coconut provides 8.1 mcg per 8-ounce serving.

THIAMINE: Also known as vitamin B1, thiamine helps the body's cells change carbohydrates into energy. Small amounts of thiamine are found in most foods, including young coconut, which contains 0.1 mg of the recommended dietary allowance of 1.1 mg for women and 1.2 mg for men.

## HEALTH BENEFITS OF GREEN COCONUT

While there are no specific studies on young green coconut, it has a long history of being used to help strengthen the sick and elderly and supply babies in coconut-producing countries with a healthy "first food." Green coconut has also been used to improve the health and appearance of skin and hair.

## CHOOSING, USING, AND KEEPING GREEN COCONUT

When you are buying whole young coconuts, avoid cracks, mold, wet spots, and discoloration. When you pick up a coconut, it should feel heavy and actually sound as if it is filled with water. While the mature, brown coconuts can be kept at room temperature, green coconuts should be refrigerated and used within five days.

To open a green coconut, use a heavy chef's knife or (even better) a cleaver. Set the coconut on a flat surface and make four deep, straight cuts, each about two inches from the coconut's pointy top. Pry the top off and pour out the water.

*Caution: If you open a coconut and discover that the water is pink or smells sour, discard it. It has gone bad.*

For recipes in this book that call for fresh coconut, use young green coconuts from your local supermarket. Unfortunately, there is no surefire way to tell how old they are, so you may end up tossing a few. It happens to me, too!

**STEPHANIE'S FAVORITE WAY TO USE GREEN COCONUT:** Blended into a tropical fruit smoothie.

### GREEN COCONUTS: DID YOU KNOW . . . ?

- The flesh of the young coconut has more fiber than the same amount of apple.
- Peak months for fresh coconuts are October through December.
- It takes twelve to thirteen months for a coconut to mature fully.
- Coconuts grow in groups containing five to twelve fruits.
- A coconut palm produces about 100 to 120 coconuts a year.
- More than twenty billion coconuts are produced each year.
- The only two states in the United States where coconuts can grow are Hawaii and Florida—and only the southern part of Florida, at that.
- A coconut will not ripen after being picked.
- Falling coconuts kill 150 people every year, 10 times the number of people killed by sharks.
- The coconut is the largest seed in the world.
- The scientific name for the coconut palm is *Cocos nucifera*.

# COCONUT WATER

Coconuts contain a large quantity of "water," filled with potassium, vitamins, and minerals. This health-supportive fluid has nourished humans for millennia. Coconut water has only recently become big business, however, and it is now popular with fitness buffs, endurance athletes, and advocates of raw food and the Paleo diet. Since coconut water first appeared in supermarkets in 2004, its popularity has not stopped climbing. According to Convenience Store News, sales increased by $400 million in the United States in 2011 alone.

While I don't personally drink huge amounts of coconut water (my husband and two of my sons adore it!), I do use it as an ingredient in coolers and smoothies. I also give it to my kids when they're down with a stomach bug, and I appreciate how it makes me feel "normal" after an intense workout or even the morning after I've celebrated a bit too enthusiastically. (Coconut water really is the best hangover remedy I've come across—not that I've had to use it too often!)

## COCONUT WATER: NUTRITION PROFILE PER SERVING (1 CUP)

**CALORIES:** 46

**FIBER:** One serving of coconut water provides 3 g of fiber to help keep your digestive tract healthy, lower blood cholesterol, and help prevent colorectal cancer.

## WHAT'S THE DIFFERENCE?

- **COCONUT WATER:** Coconut water is the clear liquid inside green coconuts. It's this liquid that you get when you buy coconut water in various kinds of packaging. Brown, mature coconuts often have a bit of watery liquid as well, but it often has a sour taste and isn't used as a beverage.

- **COCONUT MILK:** This is the liquid that comes from the grated meat of a brown coconut.

- **COCONUT FLESH:** "Flesh" is most often used to describe the almost gelatinous innards of green coconuts.

- **COCONUT MEAT:** "Meat" is what most culinary types call the creamy white innards of a brown coconut. Firm and rich, this is what many people think of when they think of coconuts. You may occasionally hear someone refer to this part of a brown coconut as "flesh," but "meat" is more commonly used.

**PROTEIN:** Protein is considered a macronutrient, which means that your body needs it in large amounts every day to perform everything from nutrient transport to cell repair. Coconut water provides 1.78 g of protein.

**AMINO ACIDS:** Coconut water contains small amounts of eighteen amino acids, which are the building blocks of protein. When digested, amino acids help the body create solid matter, including skin, eyes, heart, intestines, bones, and muscle.

**ENZYMES:** Coconut water contains enzymes, proteins that allow certain chemical reactions to take place much more quickly than they would on their own.

**VITAMIN C:** This is a water-soluble nutrient that acts as an antioxidant, helping protect cells from the damage caused by free radicals, the compounds formed when our bodies convert the food we eat into energy. A serving of coconut water provides 5.8 mg of a vitamin C.

**CALCIUM:** This mineral is necessary to maintain strong bones and healthy communication between the brain and various parts of the body. From a serving of coconut water, you'll get 58 mg of the mineral.

**COPPER:** Dietary copper is helpful in the production of red blood cells and assists with your sense of taste. While the USDA has not yet determined a daily recommended dietary allowance, it considers 2 mg an adequate daily goal for adults. A serving of coconut water provides about 96 mcg of copper.

**IRON:** While not overly abundant in iron, a serving of coconut water will give your body about 0.94 mg of the daily requirement for this mineral. Iron is necessary for cell growth, normal cellular functioning, and synthesis of some hormones and connective tissue.

**MANGANESE:** You'll get 0.3 mg of manganese, a mineral that helps you metabolize both fat and protein, from coconut water. Manganese also supports both the immune and nervous systems and promotes stable blood sugar levels.

**MAGNESIUM:** One serving of coconut water delivers about 60 mg of your daily requirement of magnesium, a mineral responsible for many biochemical functions in the body, including regulating the heart's rhythm and supporting the function of nerve cells. Magnesium is a major electrolyte that helps maintain proper fluid levels in the body and regulate muscle function.

**SELENIUM:** You'll get 60 mg of in each serving of coconut water. This nutrient plays critical roles in reproduction, thyroid hormone metabolism, DNA synthesis, and protection from oxidative damage and infection.

**SODIUM:** A mineral that is also an electrolyte, sodium helps maintain proper fluid levels in the body and regulate muscle function. There are 252 mg of sodium in a cup of coconut water.

**PHOSPHORUS:** Responsible for creating some of the energy that you use every day, phosphorus also assists your body in synthesizing proteins, fats, and carbohydrates, and regulates the fluid levels in your body. You'll get 48 mg with each serving of coconut water.

**POTASSIUM:** You'll get a whopping 600 mg of potassium in a serving of coconut water. This essential mineral, a major electrolyte, helps maintain proper fluid levels in the body and regulate muscle function. It also plays an important role in nerve function and blood pressure.

**ZINC:** Found in cells throughout the body, zinc helps the immune system fight off invading bacteria and viruses. The body also needs zinc to make proteins and DNA, the genetic material in all cells. A serving of coconut water provides 0.2 mg of the mineral.

## HEALTH BENEFITS OF COCONUT WATER

**DIABETES PREVENTION:** In the December 8, 2011, issue of the *Journal of Ethnopharmacology*, a study conducted by the Department of Pharmaceutical Technology at Jadavpur University in Kolkata, India, showed that diabetic animals that had been fed an extract of coconut water showed a significant reduction in fasting blood glucose levels compared with a diabetic control group. Other studies have shown similar results, leading to the hypothesis that coconut water might be an antidiabetic.

**ALZHEIMER'S DISEASE:** A study conducted in late 2010 by a research team from Prince of Songkla University in Hat Yai, Thailand, found that daily consumption of coconut water can help prevent the onset of Alzheimer's disease in menopausal women. Using menopausal rats, researchers studied brain abnormalities associated with Alzheimer's. After giving the rats coconut water, these abnormalities lessened considerably. Preliminary studies on young coconut juice (YCJ) have reported the presence of estrogen-like components.

**HYPERTENSION:** A 2005 study by a team from the University of the West Indies in St. Augustine, Trinidad, selected twenty-eight individuals with hypertension and divided them into three groups. Each group was assigned a specific drink; included were bottled drinking water, coconut water, and mauby fruit juice. The drinks were consumed daily for two weeks. At the end of the study, the group that received coconut water experienced a 71 percent decrease in systolic blood pressure and a 29 percent decrease in diastolic blood pressure.

**HYDRATION:** Several studies have pitted coconut water against commercially available sports drinks. For some people, coconut water seems to be a healthier alternative to these chemical-laden drinks. If you're one of them, you'll be interested in a study that was published in the *Journal of the International Society of Sports Nutrition*, January 18, 2012. Following a sixty-minute bout of dehydrating treadmill exercise, twelve exercise-trained men received bottled water, pure coconut water, coconut water from concentrate, or a carbohydrate-electrolyte sports drink on four occasions, separated by at least five days, in a random order. Hydration status (body mass, fluid retention, plasma osmolality, urine specific gravity) and performance (treadmill time to exhaustion; assessed after rehydration) were determined during the recovery period.

No differences were noted between coconut water, coconut water from concentrate, or the sports drink on any occasion. It was determined that all three beverages were capable of promoting rehydration and supporting subsequent exercise. That said, coconut water contains significantly less sodium than a leading commercial Gatorade-type sports drink. If sodium is a health concern for you, you'll find a way to create a special coconut water–based sports drink on page 55.

## CHOOSING, USING, AND KEEPING COCONUT WATER

When purchasing packaged coconut water, look at the list of ingredients. If it contains sweeteners, flavorings, and/or other additives, pass it by. You want pure, unadulterated coconut water. Always refrigerate any container of coconut water that you've opened and use it within one or two days—or freeze it for longer storage.

*Caution: You'll definitely know when coconut water is spoiled—it has a sour taste and smell.*

**STEPHANIE'S FAVORITE WAY TO USE COCONUT WATER:** To make ice cubes.

---

### COCONUT WATER: DID YOU KNOW . . . ?

- Ten years ago, the first-ever patent granted to a UN agency was awarded to the Food and Agriculture Organization (FAO) to bottle coconut water in a way that preserves its nutrients.

- Coconut water contains the same five electrolytes found in human blood. (Gatorade has only two of these electrolytes.)

- The three top-selling coconut water brands in the United States are ZICO (owned by Coca-Cola), O.N.E. (owned by Pepsi), and Vita Coco (which counts pop singer Madonna as a primary investor).

- Each coconut may contain about 200 to 1,000 mL of water depending on cultivar type and size.

- The water from coconuts that are five months old or younger tastes bitter and is low in nutrients.

- Coconut water needs to be kept out of sunlight. UV light causes coconut water to oxidize and lose nutrients.

- Coconut water is used as a supplement to breast milk in many coconut-growing countries.

- Coconut water in recipes: In the recipes in this book, I use coconut water from fresh green coconuts, or from one of several brands of no-additive, unflavored coconut water.

# MATURE COCONUT

Round, brown, and rough, with three eyes on top: That's how most of us picture coconuts. The meat of a mature coconut is white, firm, and rich—different in texture from the flesh of green coconuts, with a different nutritional profile. When removed from the shell, coconut meat can be grated or chopped and used as an ingredient—raw, cooked, baked, or frozen—in too many recipes to count, for every conceivable meal, including snacks, desserts, smoothies, juices, and treats of all kinds. Undeniably, coconut is one of nature's most versatile (and delicious) ingredients. It is an ancient staple that has nourished civilizations for thousands of years.

## MATURE COCONUT: NUTRITION PROFILE PER SERVING (1 CUP)

**CALORIES:** 283

**FIBER:** A 1-cup serving of coconut meat provides 7 g of fiber, a nutrient that helps with digestion by adding bulk to the stool, which in turn, helps move food through the digestive tract while "cleaning" the interior wall of the large intestine. Fiber has been shown to help with weight loss by creating a feeling of fullness, which discourages overeating.

**PROTEIN:** Proteins are the body's building blocks. All of our organs, including the skin, muscles, hair, and nails are built from proteins. The immune system, digestive system, and blood all rely on proteins to work correctly. You'll get 3 g of protein from a serving of coconut meat.

**MEDIUM CHAIN FATTY ACIDS:** Coconut is rich in medium chain fatty acids, which are broken down much faster than long chain fatty acids, so they provide energy, but do not contribute to high cholesterol, the way long chain fatty acids do. According to several studies, MCFAs can help lower bad cholesterol levels and increase good cholesterol levels.

**LAURIC ACID:** A monoglyceride compound, lauric acid boasts antiviral, antimicrobial, antiprotozoal, and antifungal properties. Researchers in the Philippines have even begun studies to prove the effectiveness of lauric acid against HIV/AIDS because of its strong antiviral properties. A 1-cup serving of coconut will give you 32 g of lauric acid. While there is no recommended dietary allowance for this powerful nutrient, some researchers suggest a minimum of 10 to 20 g per day.

**VITAMIN C:** Vitamin C is a powerful antioxidant that can help prevent and lessen the duration of viral illnesses, stimulate collagen production for fast wound healing, and help prevent a variety of diseases, from cancer to cataracts. A cup of coconut meat will provide a modest 2.8 g of the vitamin.

**VITAMIN E:** Another antioxidant, vitamin E helps keep the brain healthy and protects cells from the damage caused by free radicals. A serving of coconut meat provides 0.2 mg of the nutrient.

**FOLATE:** Also known as vitamin B9 or folic acid, folate helps the body make new cells. A serving of coconut meat provides 20.8 mcg.

**NIACIN:** Also known as vitamin B3, niacin is used in the body to release energy from carbohydrates and repair DNA. A serving of coconut meat provides 0.4 mg.

**PANTOTHENIC ACID:** Known as vitamin B5, pantothenic acid is essential to a wide range of chemical reactions in the body that sustain life. A serving of coconut meat will give you 2 percent of the USDA's recommended dietary allowance.

**RIBOFLAVIN:** Also known as vitamin B2, and formerly known as vitamin G, riboflavin is essential for metabolic energy production. You'll get 0.1 mg.

**THIAMINE:** Also known as vitamin B1, thiamine helps enhance brain function and keep the digestive tract healthy. You'll get 0.1 mg of the recommended dietary allowance from a cup of coconut meat.

**SELENIUM:** This mineral is essential in cell metabolism and is a powerful antioxidant that helps keep the immune system strong. A serving of coconut meat provides 8.1 mcg of the nutrient.

**CALCIUM:** This mineral is necessary to maintain strong bones and healthy communication between the brain and various parts of the body. You'll get 11.2 mg of calcium from a serving of coconut meat.

**IRON:** While not overly rich in iron, a serving of coconut will give your body 1.9 mg for this mineral. Iron is necessary for growth, development, normal cellular functioning, and synthesis of some hormones and connective tissue.

**MAGNESIUM:** Magnesium is required for the proper growth and maintenance of bones. It is also needed for the correct functioning of nerves, muscles, and many other parts of the body. A serving of coconut meat provides 25.6 mg.

**MANGANESE:** You'll get 1.2 mg of manganese, a mineral that helps you metabolize both fat and protein. Manganese also supports both the immune and nervous systems and promotes stable blood sugar levels.

**PHOSPHORUS:** After calcium, phosphorus is the second most abundant mineral in the body. It helps create strong bones and teeth. A serving of coconut meat will provide 90.4 mg of the mineral.

**POTASSIUM:** Potassium is essential for fluid balance within your cells. It is also necessary for proper heart function and muscle growth. A serving of coconut meat will provide 285 mg of potassium.

**ZINC:** Found in cells throughout the body, zinc helps the immune system fight off invading bacteria and viruses. The body also needs zinc to make proteins and DNA, the genetic material in all cells. A serving of coconut meat provides 0.9 mg of zinc.

**COPPER:** Some of the few functions of dietary copper are to help in the production of red blood cells and to assist with your sense of taste. A serving of coconut meat will provide 0.3 mg of the mineral.

## HEALTH BENEFITS OF MATURE COCONUT

**BETTER CARDIOVASCULAR HEALTH:** Before 1991, coconut was the primary dietary staple in Sri Lanka. The average Sri Lankan ate 132 coconuts per year. Heart attacks and heart disease were rare. In fact, they were so rare that in 1978 the United Nations reported that Sri Lanka had the lowest death rate from ischemic heart disease than any other country in the world. And yet, after an aggressive health campaign in the early 1990s that discouraged coconut-eating (due to a misguided theory that fat in coconut leads to heart disease), coconut consumption dropped to about 90 per person. With the drop in coconut consumption, hospital admission rates for heart attacks increased by about 120 percent for women and 137 percent for men.

A study published in the January 2012 issue of *Asia Pacific Journal of Clinical Nutrition* showed that Filipino women who consumed coconut had healthier blood lipid profiles, a major determinant of heart disease, than those who didn't.

**LOWER CHOLESTEROL LEVELS:** In a study performed by the Food and Nutrition Research Institute, in Bicutan, Taguig, in the Philippines, twenty-one test subjects with moderately elevated blood cholesterol who ate dried coconut flakes daily for fourteen weeks lowered their serum triglycerides and LDL cholesterol levels by up to 6.3 percent.

**REDUCTION OF PARASITES AND OTHER PATHOGENS:** The medium chain fatty acids and lauric acid in coconut have long been credited, in coconut-eating cultures, for their impact on reducing parasites and bacterial, fungal, and viral infections. In 2010, researchers from Heinrich Heine University in Düsseldorf, Germany, found that coconut also works to keep sheep parasite-free. Sheep with gastrointestinal nematodes and cestodes were given feed containing 60 g of coconut. After eight days, the worm stages disappeared from the feces; the sheep were still clear of the parasites at both nine and twenty days after the end of the study.

**REDUCTION OF STROKE AND HEART DISEASE RISK:** In a study published in the March 1993 issue of the *Journal of Internal Medicine,* a team of researchers from the Primary Health Care Centre in Sjöbo, Sweden, set out to study incidence of stroke in the coconut-eating population on the island of Kitava in Papua New Guinea. The population, which practices a subsistence lifestyle that is uninfluenced by Western dietary habits, relies on found tubers, fruit, fish, and coconut as dietary staples, with coconut making up the largest portion of the inhabitants' diets. Of the total population, 1,816 subjects were estimated to be older than three years of age, and 125 were estimated to be sixty to ninety-six years old. The frequencies of spontaneous sudden death, exertion-related chest pain, hemiparesis, aphasia, and sudden imbalance were assessed through semistructured interviews of 213 adults aged twenty to ninety-six. Resting electrocardiograms (ECGs) were recorded in 119 males and 52 females. No case corresponding to stroke, sudden death, or angina pectoris was described by the interviewed subjects. Stroke and heart disease were absent in this population, even in the older adults. In Western cultures, stroke and heart disease occur in an average of more than 11.3 percent of the overall, adult population.

## CHOOSING, USING, AND KEEPING MATURE COCONUT

Frozen mature coconut that has been shredded is available in some Southeast Asian and Indo-Pak groceries and has recently appeared in mainstream supermarkets (look for the Birds Eye brand) When a recipe calls for raw mature coconut meat, I prefer to do the old-fashioned thing and crack open a coconut myself.

Here's the kind of long, but very easy, way to open a mature coconut:

1. Peel away as much of the hairy fiber as you can.

2. While it is not necessary to drain the coconut before cracking, it does make things easier. To drain, insert a clean drill bit, long nail, or thin screwdriver into the softest of the three eyes on the top of the coconut. Pour any liquid into a bowl, and use immediately for cooking or making smoothies. (Discard after 24 hours; it sours quickly.)

3. To make opening easier, either freeze the coconut for a half hour before cracking or heat in a 200°F oven for 15 minutes. This is an optional step, but it will make the coconut easier to open.

4. Find the coconut's eyes. If the coconut were a globe, the eyes would be the North Pole. Look for the equator of the coconut. That's where you're going to want to tap.

5. Place the coconut in a plastic bag, if you wish, and use a hammer to tap around the equator.

6. Once the coconut cracks, pry it open and see if you can separate the white coconut meat from the shell. In many cases, you will be able to lift the meat out in large pieces.

7. With a vegetable peeler, remove any brown husk that might be stuck to the coconut meat.

### MATURE COCONUTS: DID YOU KNOW . . . ?

- The husks of mature coconuts are used in gas masks. During World War I, the United States developed a type of steam-activated coconut carbon—obtained by burning coconut husks—to use in gas masks. Masks using coconut carbon were superior at filtering noxious substances. This technology is still used today.

- Coconut-fired carbon (made from mature coconut husks) is used to clean up radiation. In fact, coconut-fired carbon was recently used to help remove radiation from the damaged Fukushima nuclear plant.

- Monkeys harvest coconuts. Not only are palm trees dangerous for humans to climb but also, it is difficult to pick a ten-pound coconut from the top of a coconut tree while holding on for dear life. That's why many coconut farmers use trained monkeys to harvest their coconuts.

- The Philippines is the world's top producer of coconuts.

- The coconut palm is also known as "the tree of life" because there are more than one hundred products that can be made from coconut palms and their fruit.

- In Southeast Asia, it is said that "he who plants a coconut tree plants food and drink, vessels and clothing, a habitation for himself, and a heritage for his children."

- The coconut may reach more than one hundred feet and has a lifetime of about seventy-five to one hundred years.

- It takes four or five years for a coconut palm to begin producing coconuts.

8. Refrigerate and use the coconut meat within a day or two, or freeze for longer storage.

*Caution: Avoid coconuts that are cracked, moldy, or weepy at the eyes. If you open a mature coconut and the meat, or any liquid, has a yellowy tint, it's spoiled—toss it and try again with a new coconut.*

(Note that a mature coconut may not contain any liquid, but if it does, it should be clear and slightly milky.) If you're not going to use it immediately, refrigerate or even freeze the unopened coconut for up to five days.

**STEPHANIE'S FAVORITE WAY TO USE MATURE COCONUT:** Eaten as-is, straight from a freshly opened coconut.

# COCONUT OIL

Coconut oil comes from the meat of mature coconuts and has been used by humans since coconuts first appeared. In coconut-producing countries, coconut oil is used as a cooking oil, food, medicine, and cosmetic; it is even used in industry. Today, most of the coconut oil we consume comes from fruit grown in coconut groves, or plantations, in Southeast Asia.

## COCONUT OIL: NUTRITION PROFILE PER SERVING (1 TABLESPOON)

**CALORIES:** 117

**MEDIUM CHAIN FATTY ACIDS:** About two-thirds of coconut oil is made up of medium chain fatty acids, known in the health world as MCFAs. In fact, coconut oil is nature's richest source of medium chain fatty acids,

## WHAT ABOUT COCONUT OIL'S UNSTUDIED BENEFITS?

There is anecdotal evidence and centuries of traditional healing wisdom that say coconut oil heals digestive disorders and soothes inflamed tissue of the large colon, helps strengthen the immune system, improves liver function, helps normalize nervous system function in children with autism and individuals with brain injuries, stabilizes blood sugar levels, helps improve bone health and lower the risk of cavities, and strengthens hair and nails. However, no research-based studies have been performed to prove any of these claims. That said, I personally believe that coconut oil can do all of these things. If you suffer from one of these conditions, why not ask your health-care provider what he or she knows about using coconut to help?

which help the body better absorb and use other nutrients, boast powerful immune-system benefits, increase metabolism for faster healing and weight loss, and assist in healing a range of health conditions from IBS to candida to cardiovascular conditions to dementia.

**LAURIC ACID:** Making up almost 50 percent of the fatty acids in coconut oil, lauric acid is known for its ability to kill a wide range of potent pathogens, including bacteria (such as staph), fungi (such as the yeast *Candida albicans*), and viruses. It also may help repair neuron and nerve function in the brain for those with Alzheimer's or brain injury or for individuals on the autistic spectrum.

**CAPRYLIC ACID:** Another fatty acid present in smaller amounts, caprylic acid is also antimicrobial. Together with lauric acid in coconut oil, caprylic acid helps increase levels of HDL cholesterol (the good cholesterol). It also helps kill bacteria, fungi (including yeast), and viruses in the body.

**PALMITIC ACID:** This fatty acid has antioxidant properties and has been shown, in animal studies, to help prevent atherosclerosis—better known as hardening, or narrowing, of the arteries.

**PHENOLIC COMPOUNDS:** The phenolic compounds found in coconut oil have antioxidant properties, and help promote healthy aging by minimizing DNA damage caused by free radicals.

# HEALTH BENEFITS OF COCONUT OIL

**IMPROVEMENT OF BLOOD CHOLESTEROL LEVELS:** Research done with both humans and rats shows that coconut oil may reduce the risk of heart disease by having favorable effects on total cholesterol, LDL cholesterol, and HDL cholesterol. Researchers at Universidade Federal de Alagoas in Brazil found that in forty women, coconut oil reduced total and LDL cholesterol to a greater degree than soybean oil, while increasing HDL to a greater degree than soybean oil. Rat studies performed at the University of Kerala, in India, have shown that coconut oil reduces triglycerides and total and LDL cholesterol, increases HDL, and improves blood coagulation factors and antioxidant status. Research at the two universities in the Netherlands, Maastricht University and Wageningen University, came upon the same conclusions.

**MEMORY IMPROVEMENT:** In a study published in the March 2014 issue of *Neurobiology of Aging*, consumption of medium chain triglycerides (MCTs) led to an immediate improvement in brain function in patients with milder forms of Alzheimer's. Two more studies—one published in the August 2009 issue of *Nutrition & Metabolism*, and the other published in *Journal of the American Society*

## MONO, MEDIUM, SATURATED—WHAT?

There are two kinds of fats found in nature: unsaturated and saturated. Unsaturated fat is typically liquid at room temperature. It's found most often in plant foods, from avocado to nuts and seeds.

Saturated fat is solid at room temperature. It is found mostly in animal foods, such as milk, cheese, and meat, and unfortunately, it can raise blood levels. A healthy diet has less than 10 percent of daily calories from saturated fat. Here, however, is where things get confusing: Coconut oil just happens to be a saturated fat, and yet it doesn't have the cholesterol-raising power of saturated fats from animal products. In fact, coconut oil—even though it is a saturated fat—can help lower harmful cholesterol.

How? The secret is in the length of the chain. Fats of all kinds are made up of fatty acids. These fatty acids are chains of carbon and hydrogen atoms. Fats with short chains are called short chain fatty acids, or SCFAs. These are found in large quantities in dairy products.

Fats with long chain fatty acids are known as LCFAs and are found most often in the skin and organs and muscle tissues of animals. Probably 98 to 100 percent of all the fats we eat consist of LCT.

Fats with medium chain fatty acids are called MCFAs. Coconut oil is one of the only foods around that is composed mostly of medium chain fatty acids, though they also exist in palm kernel oil. MCFAs are more easily digested and used by the body than long chain fatty acids; also they help the body metabolize other nutrients more efficiently, as well as use them for energy more readily.

Just to confuse you a bit further: Sometimes you'll see these chains referred to as SCT, LCT, or MCT. The "T" stands for "triglyceride," a molecule made up mostly of fatty acids.

*for Experimental NeuroTherapeutics* July 2008 issue—found that the fatty acids in coconut oil can increase energy to the brain cells of Alzheimer's patients and relieve symptoms.

**IMPROVED METABOLISM AND BURNING OF CALORIES:** The medium chain triglycerides in coconut oil have been shown to increase twenty-four-hour energy expenditure by as much as 5 percent, potentially leading to significant weight loss over the long term. A 1996 study performed by the University of Geneva in Switzerland found that consuming about 15 to 30 g of MCTs per day increased twenty-four-hour energy expenditure by 5 percent, totaling about 120 calories per day. Research performed at the University of Naples Federico II in Italy, in 1991, concluded that calorie burning was increased in research subjects of any size after consuming medium chain fatty acids.

**KILLING OF PATHOGENS:** In clinical research and studies performed by a wide range of universities, the lauric acid and other fatty acids in coconut oil have been found helpful in preventing infections on the skin and in the body. How? By killing harmful pathogens on and in the body, including those caused by bacteria, fungi (such as yeasts), and viruses. Among these are staph and candida.

**FIGHTS VIRAL CONDITIONS:** According to a study led by Dr. Gilda Sapphire Erguiza, a pediatric pulmonologist at the Philippine Children's Medical Center in Quezon City, children with pneumonia who were treated with antibiotics and coconut oil benefited more than those taking the antibiotics alone.

**REDUCTION OF APPETITE TO HELP WEIGHT LOSS:** Several studies have found that medium chain fatty acids (MCFAs)—like the ones in coconut oil—have been found to reduce appetite, which may help with weight loss and weight maintenance. A 1996 study by researchers at the Rowett Institute of Nutrition and Health in Aberdeen, Scotland, found that men who ate the most MCFAs consumed 256 fewer calories per day, on average, than their counterparts eating a typical Western diet. A 1998 study at Institut Européen des Sciences in Dijon, France, discovered that men who ate the most MCFAs at breakfast ate significantly fewer calories at lunch.

**REDUCTION OF BELLY FAT:** Coconut oil appears to be especially effective in reducing fat in the abdominal cavity and around organs. This is the most dangerous fat of all and is highly associated with many modern-day diseases. Research conducted by the Universidade Federal de Alagoas in Brazil in 2009 on forty women with abdominal obesity found that supplementing their diet with 30 mL (1 ounce) of coconut oil per day led to a significant reduction in both body mass index (BMI) and waist circumference in twelve weeks. A 2011 study performed by Universiti Sains Malaysia on twenty obese males discovered a reduction in waist circumference of 2.86 cm (1.1 inches) after four weeks of ingesting 30 mL (1 ounce) of coconut oil per day.

**HEALING AND PROTECTION OF SKIN:** Researchers at Makati Medical Center in Makati City, Philippines, found that coconut oil was superior to mineral oil–based moisturizers in healing rough, dry, itchy skin. Researchers at the University of Belgrade in Serbia recently found that in test subjects, coconut oil applied topically blocked 20 percent of the sun's ultraviolet rays.

# CHOOSING, USING, AND KEEPING COCONUT OIL

**USE COLD-PRESSED VIRGIN COCONUT OIL:** While there are many ways of extracting this oil—from using chemicals to heat—the most traditional method is cold-pressing. This involves literally pressing the oil from the coconut using physical force (sometimes the coconut meat is soaked in water before being pressed, called "wet-milled"). Cold-pressing preserves all of coconut oil's nutrient profile. The term "virgin" (or the infrequently used "extra-virgin"—the two names mean the same thing in the coconut oil industry) refers to how many times the coconut meat has been pressed. This terminology was originally created for olive oil, but is commonly used in the coconut oil world as well. Virgin coconut oil comes from the first pressing. This is what you want.

**WHAT ABOUT ORGANIC?** Pesticides are sometimes used on nonorganic coconut palms. Not all coconut growers can afford to apply for organic certification. And not all coconut growers are interested in applying for organic certification. A 2008 study published in *Extensions du domaine de l'analyse* (vol. 17, no. 2) by researchers from the Netherlands looked at pesticide residue percentages from 2003 to 2007 in coconut oil from the Philippines. They found no pesticide residue. I personally am more concerned if the oil is cold-pressed and virgin than I am with the organic label. However, organic, cold-pressed, virgin coconut oil does exist!

**PREPARING FOOD WITH COCONUT OIL:** Coconut oil is a fine choice for baking, popping corn, or sautéing. It's equally good enjoyed in a room temperature salad dressing or a frozen dessert.

**STORING COCONUT OIL IS EASY:** Place it in the fridge if you want it to be solid. Place it in a cupboard if you like it to be more liquid. To extend its shelf life, I personally would not keep it near an oven or stove, but I know people who do and haven't experienced any rancid oil. Because of its high antioxidant content, coconut oil takes years to go rancid. Use your coconut oil up within two or three years and you should be fine.

*Caution: I cannot tell a lie: Coconut oil is a high-calorie food. As noted in the nutrition profile provided earlier, 1 tablespoon has 117 calories. I give my very skinny sons several tablespoons a day. I limit myself to 1 tablespoon on most days. Some days I go a bit crazy and have 1 ½ tablespoons.*

**COCONUT OIL IN RECIPES:** I used a variety of brands of coconut oil in the recipes in this book. When I call for "liquid coconut oil," I do not mean coconut oil that has been treated with chemicals or chemically altered to keep it liquid. I mean plain old cold-pressed virgin coconut oil that has sat in a place long enough for it to become liquid. When I call for semisolid oil, I mean the same oil, placed in the fridge for a while to harden it up a bit. Easy, safe, healthy.

**STEPHANIE'S FAVORITE WAYS TO USE COCONUT OIL:** To make popcorn, or to make a fast face scrub by mixing coconut oil with an equal amount of sugar.

# COCONUT BUTTER

Coconut butter is a lovely, luxurious way to enjoy the meat of the mature coconut. It is simply dried coconut that has been pulverized into a creamy spread—sometimes with a bit of coconut oil, but usually not. Try making your own by tossing a handful of dried unsweetened coconut into your food processor and pulsing until it becomes a paste. This wonderful food can be whipped with sweetener and used as frosting, thinned with coconut milk and coconut nectar for a dessert sauce, spread on bread and waffles, and stirred into sauces or anything else you want to do with it.

## COCONUT BUTTER: NUTRITION PROFILE PER SERVING (1 TABLESPOON)

**CALORIES:** 100

**FIBER:** A serving of coconut butter offers 2 g of fiber to help promote weight loss by creating a feeling of fullness, while encouraging efficient digestion as well. Fiber has also been found to lower the risk of certain cancers, such as colorectal cancer and other gastrointestinal cancers.

**PROTEIN:** With 2 g of protein per tablespoon, coconut butter is an easy way to increase the protein in your diet. Protein is the macronutrient responsible for helping your body build and repair itself.

**AMINO ACIDS:** Amino acids make up protein in food. When digested, they help the body create solid matter, including skin, eyes, heart, intestines, bones, and muscle. Depending upon which nutrition scientist you ask, there are between twenty and twenty-two amino acids. Of those, eight to ten are considered essential, meaning you must get these from your diet, as your body can't synthesize them from other materials.

**MEDIUM CHAIN FATTY ACIDS:** Like other coconut products, coconut butter boasts large amounts of medium chain fatty acids. MCFAs have shown promise in regulating blood sugar, helping brain function, reducing abdominal obesity, and diminishing fat storage.

**LAURIC ACID:** Coconut butter contains lauric acid, which is known for its bacteria- and virus-killing properties. It is the same acid that is found in breast milk and helps boost newborns' immunity, protecting them against infections.

**IRON:** While not overly rich in iron, a serving of coconut butter will give your body about 0.4 mg for this mineral. Iron is necessary for growth, development, normal cellular functioning, and synthesis of some hormones and connective tissue.

**MANGANESE:** One serving of coconut butter offers 0.4 mg of manganese, a mineral that the body needs to process cholesterol, carbohydrates, and protein.

## HEALTH BENEFITS OF COCONUT BUTTER

Because coconut butter is made from dried coconut meat, any of the studies on dried coconut apply to coconut butter. One of these, undertaken in 2004 by a team from the Food and Nutrition Research Institute in Bicutan, Taguig, in the Philippines, found that after fourteen weeks of eating dried flaked coconut daily, twenty-one adult men and women with moderately high blood cholesterol levels reduced their LDL cholesterol and serum triglycerides by an average of 20 percent.

## CHOOSING, USING, AND KEEPING COCONUT BUTTER

Look for coconut butter that contains whole coconut only, or whole coconut and coconut oil. Avoid any brands that contain sweeteners or additives. Once you bring it home, it will stay soft and spreadable if kept at room temperature, where it should be fine for up to a year. For longer storage, stash in your fridge and soften it up by allowing it to come to room temperature before using.

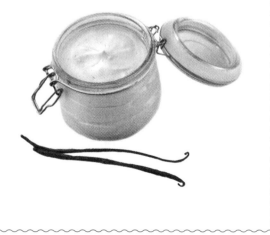

*Caution: As coconut products get more popular and more companies rush to get in on the action, new ways are created to sell coconut. You can even find coconut butter flavored with chocolate. Yes, it sounds yummy, doesn't it? But this isn't a healthful product. If you want to get it and call it dessert, be my guest, but don't be deceived: Sweetened coconut butter ("even" with chocolate) is not a health food.*

**COCONUT BUTTER IN RECIPES:** All of the recipes in this book that include coconut butter were tested using thick, homemade coconut butter and Nutiva brand Coconut Manna coconut butter.

**STEPHANIE'S FAVORITE WAY TO USE COCONUT BUTTER:** As a spread for toast and waffles.

# COCONUT MILK

Coconut milk is a delicious, milky beverage that is created when mature coconut meat (either dried or not) is ground together with water and then allowed to sit for a bit to develop its flavor. Afterward, the solids are strained away. Coconut milk is an essential ingredient in Pacific Island and Southeast Asian cooking. In the Western world, coconut milk was relegated to a dessert ingredient until the last five or six years. Now it is commonly used as a dairy-free milk for people who need to remove dairy products from their diet, and for children who are on the autistic spectrum and who are thought to react to the casein in dairy milk.

Canned coconut milk is still the most popular option around. But there are other excellent options, including frozen coconut milk, coconut milk beverage boxes and cartons (these are typically thinned with water and treated with various emulsifiers, flavorings, and stabilizers), and dried coconut milk that can be mixed with water. According to research presented at the United Nations Conference on Trade and Development, coconut milk accounts for 30 percent of coconut products sold worldwide.

## COCONUT MILK: NUTRITION PROFILE PER SERVING (¼ CUP)

**CALORIES:** 100

**MEDIUM CHAIN FATTY ACIDS:** Unlike long chain fatty acids, MCFAs are easily and quickly metabolized into energy in the liver. It is believed that because MCFAs are used more quickly by the body than other types of fatty acids, they are less likely to be stored as fat.

**LAURIC ACID:** Antiviral and antibacterial, lauric acid destroys a wide variety of disease-causing organisms. It may also reduce cholesterol and triglyceride levels, which lowers heart disease and risk of stroke.

**FIBER:** One serving of coconut milk provides 1.6 g of fiber to help keep your digestive tract healthy.

**PROTEIN:** Protein is considered a macronutrient, which means that your body needs it in large amounts every day to perform everything from nutrient transport to cell repair. Coconut milk provides just under 2 g per serving.

**IRON:** The mineral iron is a part of all cells and does many things in our bodies such as delivering oxygen to our blood. One serving of coconut milk provides 1.875 mg of iron.

**VITAMIN C:** Vitamin C is a water-soluble nutrient that acts as an antioxidant in the body, helping to protect cells from the damage caused by free radicals, the compounds formed when our bodies convert the food we eat into energy. A quarter-cup serving of coconut milk provides 2 percent of the daily requirement.

**VITAMIN E:** Vitamin E is a fat-soluble nutrient that also acts as an antioxidant, helping protect cells from the damage caused by free radicals.

**NIACIN:** A serving of coconut milk provides .456 mg of vitamin B3, also known as niacin. Niacin helps reduce atherosclerosis, or hardening of the arteries. For people who have already had a heart attack, niacin seems to lower the risk of a second one. It also helps lower the risk of Alzheimer's disease, cataracts, osteoarthritis, and type 1 diabetes.

**FOLATE:** Folate is a B vitamin that is naturally present in many foods. (In case you ever wondered, folate and folic acid are forms of the same B vitamin. Folate occurs naturally in food, and folic acid is the synthetic form of this vitamin.) The body needs folate to make DNA and other genetic material. Folate is also needed for the body's cells to divide. A serving of coconut milk provides 8 percent of the daily requirement.

**SELENIUM:** You'll get 3.72 mcg of selenium in each serving of coconut milk. This nutrient plays critical roles in reproduction, thyroid hormone metabolism, DNA synthesis, and protection from oxidative damage and infection.

**POTASSIUM:** You'll get 158 mg of potassium in one serving of coconut milk. This essential mineral is a major electrolyte found in the human body. In addition, it plays an important role in electrolyte regulation, nerve function, muscle control, and blood pressure.

**PHOSPHORUS:** Phosphorus is responsible for creating some of the energy that you use every day. It also assists your body in synthesizing proteins, fats, and carbohydrates and regulates the fluid levels in your body. You'll get 60 mg with each serving of coconut milk.

**MAGNESIUM:** One serving of coconut milk delivers about 25 mg of magnesium, a mineral responsible for many biochemical functions in the body, including regulating the heart's rhythm and supporting the function of nerve cells.

## HEALTH BENEFITS OF COCONUT MILK

**REVS UP YOUR METABOLISM:** Two small studies, one conducted in Italy with eight men, and one in Switzerland with twelve men, showed that individuals who ate meals that contained about 30 g of medium chain fatty acids had a roughly 5 percent higher metabolic rate compared to those who ate long chain fatty acids. One cup of coconut milk has around 34 g of MFCAs.

**BURNS MORE CALORIES:** Researchers from McGill University in Canada published the results of their MCFA study in the *American Journal of Clinical Nutrition* in 1999. Twelve women were fed meals enriched with either MCFAs from butter and coconut oil or LCFAs from beef fat. After fourteen days, the women who ate the MCFA-rich food were burning about 33 more calories per minute than the women who had eaten the LCFA meals.

**SPEEDS WEIGHT LOSS:** In a sixteen-week study published in the *American Journal of Clinical Nutrition* in 2008, researchers fed forty men and women meals that contained the same number of calories, but contained either long chain fatty acids or medium chain fatty acids, the type of fat found in coconut. Those who ate the MCFA-rich meals lost an average of 6.6 pounds, whereas those who ate the LCFA-laden meals lost 3.3 pounds.

## CHOOSING, USING, AND KEEPING COCONUT MILK

Be careful to check the "use by" date, and look for any damage—dents, for example—in cans of coconut milk. Once opened, transfer the contents to a resealable container and refrigerate. Use the milk within a few days. The high oil content in coconut milk can make it turn rancid if it is not stored under proper conditions.

*Caution: If you are concerned with bisphenol A (BPA)—a chemical used in the lining of certain canned foods—you may want to look for coconut milk in BPA-free cans or aseptic boxes. BPA can leach into foods that are acidic (such as tomato products) or fatty (such as coconut milk). BPA has been linked to cancer, asthma, diabetes, and impaired neurological development. It has also been shown to impact the body's natural response to estrogen, leading to a wide variety of hormonal imbalances.*

**COCONUT MILK IN RECIPES:** In recipes where coconut milk is called for, I use canned regular coconut milk (not "lite"), and preferably without a stabilizer such as guar gum. (If "lite" is all you can find, go ahead and use it.) Coconut milk in boxes and cartons has added water, thickeners, colorants, preservatives, emulsifiers, and other ingredients that aren't good for you, and that can change the character of the recipe. There are a few recipes in the book, however, where it is fine to use coconut milk from a box or carton. (These are all clearly marked.)

**STEPHANIE'S FAVORITE WAY TO USE COCONUT MILK:** I use coconut milk daily as a replacement for dairy milk. I can't think of a way that I don't use it!

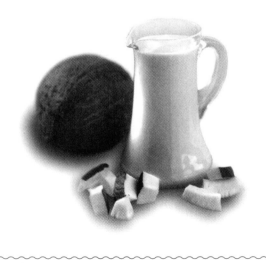

# COCONUT CREAM

Coconut cream is very similar to coconut milk but contains less water. The difference is mainly consistency. Coconut cream has a thicker, more paste-like consistency, while coconut milk is generally a liquid. Commercial coconut milks and creams are generally sold in cans, although some are sold in boxes and Tetra Paks. The main ingredient in these products is water. If the fat content is 17 percent, it is called "coconut milk." If the fat content is 24 percent, it is called "coconut cream."

## COCONUT CREAM: NUTRITION PROFILE PER SERVING (1 TABLESPOON)

**CALORIES:** Around 50

**PROTEIN:** With a very modest 1 g of protein per serving, coconut cream provides some of the macronutrient responsible for helping your body build and repair itself.

**MEDIUM CHAIN FATTY ACIDS:** Coconut products, including coconut cream, are among the world's most concentrated sources of medium chain fatty acids, which help the body better absorb and use other nutrients. Coconut creams boast powerful immune-system benefits while increasing metabolism for faster healing and weight loss, and they help heal a range of health conditions from IBS and candida to cardiovascular conditions and dementia.

**LAURIC ACID:** Lauric acid makes up almost 50 percent of the fatty acids in coconut products, including coconut cream. It is known for its ability to kill a wide range of potent pathogens, including bacteria (such as staph), fungi (such as the yeast *Candida albicans*), and viruses.

**IRON:** The body must have iron to help it create red blood cells. Coconut cream contains just a tiny bit of the recommended 8 mg.

## COCONUT CREAM VS. CREAM OF COCONUT

Coconut cream is a very thick, paste-like cream—a concentrate, in essence, where most of the water has been removed. To make coconut cream, the first step is to chill coconut milk and then skim off the rich layer of cream that forms on top.

Cream of coconut is a canned, sweetened product, typically found in the same aisle as premade drink mixes and drink syrups. I think of it as the coconut-based version of condensed sweetened milk. Most brands of cream of coconut have a photo of a piña colada or other frozen drink on the front of the can. Cream of coconut is coconut cream that has been cooked with corn syrup or sugar, and it is a popular ingredient in sweet coconut-flavored "tropical" mixed drinks.

# HEALTH BENEFITS OF COCONUT CREAM

**ANTIULCER:** While there have been no dedicated studies using coconut cream, there have been plenty involving coconut milk, a product with almost identical—though more diluted—ingredients than coconut cream. One surprising study involved a large group of rats with ulcers. Split into three subgroups, one group was given 40 mg of the ulcer-treating medication indomethacin each day. Another was fed 2 mL of coconut milk every day. And the last group received 2 mL of coconut water each day. The group given medication and the group given coconut milk experienced a 54 percent reduction in ulcers. The coconut water group experienced a 39 percent reduction. If you suffer from ulcers or are prone to them, coconut cream and coconut milk may be helpful additions to your daily diet.

# CHOOSING, USING, AND KEEPING COCONUT CREAM

treat coconut cream just as you would coconut milk: Store it in a cupboard or pantry until you open it and refrigerate any unused portion. Use the remainder within two days of opening the container. Freeze coconut cream for longer storage.

*Caution: Avoid buying cream of coconut, a heavily sweetened, processed, syrupy, coconut milk product.*

**COCONUT CREAM IN RECIPES:** In recipes where coconut cream is called for, I use both Native Forest and Trader Joe's brands interchangeably. Trader Joe's brand is richer, but both work well.

**STEPHANIE'S FAVORITE WAY TO USE COCONUT CREAM:** To make whipped cream to top berry desserts.

# COCONUT FLOUR

Coconut flour is today's darling in the culinary world. The gluten-free crowd loves it for the way it adds moisture to typically dry wheat-free baked goods. Paleo eaters adore its low-carb, high-protein profile. Healthy types love how easy it is to add brain-gut-immune-system-healing medium chain fatty acids and lauric acid to foods by using coconut flour, and the rest of us just love the taste.

For those of you who are not familiar with coconut flour, it is a delicious by-product of coconut oil and coconut milk: To make coconut oil, coconut is dry-pressed using heat to help extract the oil. Or, it is soaked in water and then pressed for its oil. The remaining pulp is then dried and ground into flour. This is what is meant when people say that coconut flour has been defatted. I encourage you to read more about coconut flour and then give it a try! In this book, there are loads of recipes with coconut flour just waiting for you to enjoy them!

## COCONUT FLOUR: NUTRITION PROFILE PER SERVING (2 TABLESPOONS)

**CALORIES:** 120

**MEDIUM CHAIN FATTY ACIDS:** Unlike long chain fatty acids, MCFAs are easily and quickly metabolized into energy in the liver. It is believed that they are less likely to be stored as fat because they are used more quickly by the body than other types of fatty acids.

**LAURIC ACID:** Antiviral and antibacterial, lauric acid destroys a wide variety of disease-causing organisms. It may also reduce cholesterol and triglyceride levels, thereby lowering heart disease and risk of stroke.

**FIBER:** One serving of coconut flour provides 11 g of fiber to help maintain a healthy digestive tract.

**PROTEIN:** Protein is considered a macronutrient, which means that your body needs it in large amounts every day to perform everything from nutrient transport to cell repair. Two tablespoons of coconut flour provides 2 g.

**IRON:** The mineral iron is a part of all cells and does many things in our bodies, including delivering oxygen to blood. Two tablespoons of coconut flour provides about 5 g.

**SODIUM:** A mineral that is also an electrolyte, sodium helps maintain proper fluid levels in the body and regulates muscle function. You'll get 56 g per serving of coconut flour.

## COCONUT FLOUR: DID YOU KNOW . . . ?

- Coconut flour has about 1 g of healthy fat per tablespoon.

- Coconut flour has about 2.5 g of fiber per tablespoon.

- Coconut flour absorbs huge amounts of water, which can help keep foods soft and chewy. Even if you bake with traditional wheat flours, using a couple of tablespoons of coconut flour helps tenderize pie dough and shortbread and helps keep baked goods fresh. If you'd like to try using coconut flour to improve the keeping quality of most mainstream recipes, swap in 10 to 15 percent coconut flour for any wheat-based flours.

- Because coconut flour has been defatted, it's leaner than other nut flours. It cannot be used as a substitute for any type of nut meal or nut-based flour, however.

- Coconut flour has about 61 percent fiber in its makeup compared to 27 percent in wheat flour.

## HEALTH BENEFITS OF COCONUT FLOUR

**HELPS REDUCE RISK OF SKIN CANCER:** A 1997 study performed by a team at Annamalai University in Annamalai Nagar, India, found that when rats with skin cancers were fed coconut flour, they had fewer lesions, tumors, and cancerous cells than rats that were fed red chili pepper.

**LOWERS BLOOD CHOLESTEROL:** A study published in the August 1998 issue of the *Indian Journal of Experimental Biology* followed rats that were fed a diet of hemicellulose fiber–rich coconut flour and another group fed a fiber-free diet. (Note: Rather than just long straight chains like cellulose fiber, hemicellulose may have side chains and branches. Both types of fiber are found in fruits, veggies, and legumes.) The rats that ate the hemicellulose-coconut diet showed decreased concentration of total cholesterol and increased HDL cholesterol (the healthy kind), while the fiber-free group showed no change.

## CHOOSING, USING, AND KEEPING COCONUT FLOUR

Coconut flour absorbs large amounts of liquid. When baking with it, opt for recipes that have been developed for coconut flour, or substitute no more than 10 percent to 15 percent of the flour in a standard recipe with coconut flour. Because it is often clumpy, vigorously whisk coconut flour before using it to get the lumps out. Coconut flour does not go rancid quickly, but if you're like me, it takes a while to use up a whole bag of the stuff. To keep it fresh, store it in an airtight container in the freezer.

*Caution: Coconut flour should smell and taste mild and rich, and have a very subtle coconut flavor. If it tastes rancid or off, toss it.*

**COCONUT FLOUR IN RECIPES:** All of the recipes in this book that use coconut flour were tested using several brands. Note: Calories and nutrient contents differ— sometimes greatly—between brands.

**STEPHANIE'S FAVORITE WAY TO USE COCONUT FLOUR:** I love adding a few tablespoons of coconut flour to non–coconut flour recipes to create extra moistness and increase the longevity of baked goods.

# DRIED COCONUT

Dried flaked coconut, often called desiccated coconut, is a worldwide favorite. It is a whole food, made by drying the meat of mature coconuts. It's typically sold in flakes of different widths, from a wide flake to the finest of flakes (called macaroon coconut). While you may be familiar with the sweetened, slightly sticky "Angel Flake" coconut found in the baking aisle of most supermarkets, make an effort to search out unadulterated dried coconut. It's delicious, easy to cook with, and nutritious. In fact, it has a similar nutritional profile to coconut meat.

## DRIED COCONUT: NUTRITION PROFILE PER SERVING (2 TABLESPOONS)

**CALORIES:** 185

**FIBER:** A serving of dried coconut provides 8 g of fiber, a nutrient that helps with digestion by adding bulk to the stool, which helps move food through the digestive tract and "clean" the interior wall of the large intestine. Fiber can help with weight loss by creating a feeling of fullness, which discourages overeating.

**PROTEIN:** Proteins are the body's building blocks. All of our organs, including the skin, muscles, hair, and nails, are built from proteins. The immune system, digestive system, and blood all rely on proteins to work correctly. You'll get 2 g from a serving of dried coconut.

**MEDIUM CHAIN FATTY ACIDS:** Dried coconut is rich in medium chain fatty acids, which are broken down much faster than long chain fatty acids, so they provide energy but do not contribute to high cholesterol, as long chain fatty acids do. According to several studies, MCFAs can help lower bad cholesterol levels and increase good cholesterol levels.

**LAURIC ACID:** Dried coconut is rich in lauric acid, a monoglyceride compound that exhibits antiviral, antimicrobial, antiprotozoal, and antifungal properties. Because of its strong antiviral properties, studies have begun in the Philippines attempting to prove the effectiveness of lauric acid against HIV/AIDS.

**VITAMIN B6:** The body uses vitamin B6 for more than one hundred enzyme reactions involved in metabolism. B6 is also involved in brain development and immune function in utero and during infancy. A serving of dried coconut will give you 4 percent of the recommended dietary allowance.

**VITAMIN C:** Vitamin C is a powerful antioxidant that can stimulate collagen production for fast wound healing, help prevent and lessen the duration of viral illnesses, and help prevent a variety of other diseases, from cancer to cataracts. A serving of dried coconut will give you 0.1 mg.

**VITAMIN E:** Another antioxidant, vitamin E helps keep the brain healthy. It also protects cells from the damage caused by free radicals. A serving of dried coconut provides 1 percent of the recommended dietary allowance.

**FOLATE:** Also known as vitamin B9 or folic acid, folate helps the body make new cells. A serving of dried coconut provides 2.5 mcg of the recommended dietary allowance.

**PANTOTHENIC ACID:** Known as vitamin B5, pantothenic acid is essential to a wide range of chemical reactions in the body that sustain life. A serving of dried coconut provides 0.2 mg.

**RIBOFLAVIN:** Also known as vitamin B2, and formerly known as vitamin G, riboflavin is essential for metabolic energy production. You'll get 0.1 mg of the recommended dietary allowance from a serving of dried coconut.

**CALCIUM:** This mineral is necessary to maintain strong bones and healthy communication between the brain and various parts of the body. You'll get 7.38 mg of calcium.

**COPPER:** Dietary copper plays a small role in the production of red blood cells and assists with your sense of taste. A serving of dried coconut provides 0.2 mg.

**IRON:** While not overly rich in iron, a serving of dried coconut gives the body 0.9 g. This mineral is necessary for growth, development, normal cellular functioning, and synthesis of some hormones and connective tissue.

**MAGNESIUM:** Magnesium is required for the proper growth and maintenance of bones. It is also required for the proper function of nerves, muscles, and many other parts of the body. A serving of dried coconut provides 25.2 mg of the recommended dietary allowance.

**MANGANESE:** From one serving of dried coconut, you'll get 0.8 mg of manganese, a mineral that helps you metabolize both fat and protein. Manganese also supports both the immune and nervous systems and promotes stable blood sugar levels.

**PHOSPHORUS:** The body uses phosphorus to create strong bones—in fact, 85 percent of the phosphorus in the human body is found in the bones. A serving of dried coconut will provide 57.7 mg of the recommended dietary allowance.

**POTASSIUM:** Potassium is essential for fluid balance within your cells. It is also necessary for proper heart function and muscle growth. A serving of dried coconut provides 152 mg of the mineral.

**SELENIUM:** This mineral is essential in cell metabolism and is a powerful antioxidant that helps keep the immune system strong. A serving of dried coconut provides 5.2 mcg.

**ZINC:** Found in cells throughout the body, zinc helps the immune system fight off invading bacteria and viruses. The body also needs zinc to make proteins and DNA, the genetic material in all cells. A serving of dried coconut provides 0.6 mg.

## HEALTH BENEFITS OF DRIED COCONUT

**LOWERS RISK OF COLON CANCER:** An animal study performed in 2014 by a team from Annamalai University in Annamalai Nagar, India, found that eating dried coconut for thirty weeks "significantly decreased the incidence and number of tumors as well as the activity of cancerous cells" in thirty rats with colon cancer.

**LOWERS BLOOD CHOLESTEROL:** After reviewing all available research, a team at the University of Kerala, in Thiruvananthapuram, Kerala, India, concluded that eating dried coconut with coconut oil reduced serum total and LDL cholesterol in humans with high cholesterol better than coconut oil alone. This was also found in separate research performed on rats.

## CHOOSING, USING, AND KEEPING DRIED COCONUT

Dried coconut is fun to use. You'll find it in a regular medium-size shred, as well as in a finely shredded version, sometimes called macaroon coconut. I've even seen ultrawide shreds, which are a fun, chewy addition to granola and trail mix. The only thing I'd ask you to watch for is the ingredient list on packaging: Make sure you're buying a product without sweeteners and chemical preservatives. You can keep dried coconut on a dark, dry, cool shelf, but it will last longer in the refrigerator or freezer.

*Caution: To avoid rancidity, store dried coconut in the freezer or fridge and use it within a year.*

**DRIED COCONUT IN RECIPES:** All recipes in this book that use dried coconut were tested using a variety of brands of unsweetened shredded dried coconut.

**STEPHANIE'S FAVORITE WAY TO USE DRIED COCONUT:** As a breading for fish and poultry.

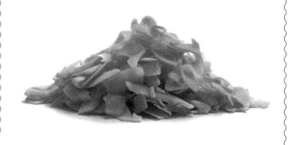

# COCONUT YOGURT

Once upon a time, all yogurt was made of cow, sheep, or goat milk, and you either ate it or you didn't. If you didn't digest lactose or if casein caused neurological problems or if you just didn't like the foggy way you felt after eating dairy, then you avoided it. Today things are different. People who choose not to consume dairy have plenty of great options, including yogurt made with coconut milk. Several companies make coconut yogurt and call it either "coconut milk yogurt" or "cultured coconut milk." It is available unsweetened, unflavored, and "Greek style." You can also make your own by fermenting coconut milk with yogurt starter.

## COCONUT YOGURT (UNFLAVORED, UNSWEETENED): NUTRITION PROFILE PER SERVING (4-OUNCE CONTAINER)

**CALORIES:** 80

**FIBER:** A serving of unflavored regular coconut yogurt contains 3 g of fiber, which promotes normal digestion, helps remove toxins from the body, and creates a feeling of fullness, which helps prevent overeating.

**PROBIOTICS:** The normal human digestive tract contains about four hundred types of probiotic bacteria that reduce the growth of harmful bacteria and promote a healthy digestive system. Fermented foods are rich in these helpful probiotics. Coconut yogurt—like its dairy counterpart—is no exception and can help reduce infections in the digestive tract, prevent (or recover from) diarrhea, and control inflammation.

**MEDIUM CHAIN FATTY ACIDS:** Medium chain fatty acids help the body absorb and use other nutrients. In addition, they boast powerful immune-system benefits, increase metabolism for faster healing and weight loss, and assist in healing a range of health conditions from IBS to candida to cardiovascular conditions to dementia.

**CALCIUM:** Because coconut milk contains only a small amount of calcium—and in order to compete with dairy yogurt—most commercial brands of coconut yogurt are fortified with calcium. Thus, a 4-ounce container of fortified regular, unflavored coconut yogurt provides about 250 mg of calcium, a mineral needed to maintain strong bones and carry out many other important functions. Almost all calcium is stored in bones and teeth, where it supports structure and hardness. The body also needs calcium for muscles to move and for nerves to carry messages between the brain and every other part of the body.

**VITAMIN B12:** Although coconut milk does not contain vitamin B12, most commercially available coconut yogurt is enriched with the vitamin. Thus, a 4-ounce container of unflavored coconut yogurt contains 1.5 mcg of vitamin B12. This nutrient is needed to keep the body's nerve and blood cells healthy and helps make DNA, the genetic material in all cells.

**MAGNESIUM:** Coconut milk—and by extension, coconut yogurt—is a magnesium-rich food. A serving of coconut yogurt provides about 80 mg of magnesium, a mineral needed for many processes in the body, including regulating muscle and nerve function, blood sugar levels, and blood pressure, as well as making protein, bone, and DNA.

**IRON:** A serving of coconut yogurt offers 0.75 mg of iron, a mineral used by the body to create red blood cells.

## HEALTH BENEFITS OF COCONUT YOGURT

**WEIGHT CONTROL:** Much of the fat in coconut yogurt is in the form of medium chain fatty acids, which can help control weight, according to a joint study in 2001 by a team from the Division of Healthcare Science Research Laboratory in Kanagawa, Japan; Kagawa Nutrition University in Saitama, Japan; and the Institute of

---

### YOGURT DEFINED

The word "yogurt" is derived from Turkish *yoğurt*, and is related to the Turkish verb *yoğurmak*, which means to be curdled, coagulated, or thickened.

---

Environmental Science for Human Life, in Tokyo. In a twelve-week, double-blind study using seventy-eight men and women, both groups were fed the same diet each day, but only one of the groups was given long chain fatty acids daily. The other was given medium chain fatty acids. It was found that the group that consumed medium chain fatty acids saw a decrease in blood cholesterol, and in body fat and weight, with an increase in metabolism.

## CHOOSING, USING, AND KEEPING COCONUT YOGURT

Coconut yogurt is available in the dairy case at health food stores, and even the most mainstream supermarkets, right next to traditional dairy yogurt. Flavored and unflavored coconut yogurt is available in both regular and thick Greek styles. Store coconut yogurt in the fridge, as you would dairy yogurt, and use it before the expiration date. Coconut yogurt can be used as a direct substitute in recipes that call for dairy yogurt, or you can whisk it with a bit of sweetener to make a quick dessert sauce.

*Caution: I am not a fan of flavored yogurts. Most of them provide more sugar in one sitting than you need, from 13 to 24 g! This is especially harmful to anyone who has blood sugar issues or suffers from sugar-induced cravings. If you're going to use coconut milk yogurt, keep it healthy by sticking to the unflavored varieties and dress it up with your own fruit, nuts, and other add-ins.*

**COCONUT YOGURT IN RECIPES:** All recipes in this book that use coconut yogurt were tested using commercially available unflavored regular coconut yogurt.

**STEPHANIE'S FAVORITE WAYS TO USE COCONUT YOGURT:** In baked goods and other recipes that call for dairy yogurt.

# COCONUT KEFIR

Kefir dates back many centuries to the shepherds of the Caucasus Mountains, who carried milk stored in leather pouches, where it would ferment into fizzy, sour yogurt. These days, confusingly enough, coconut kefir can be one of two things: a fermented coconut milk drink or a fermented coconut water drink. You will see both in markets and online.

## COCONUT KEFIR: NUTRITION PROFILE PER SERVING (1 CUP)

**CALORIES:** 70 in a serving of coconut milk kefir; around 10 in a serving of coconut water kefir.

**PROBIOTICS:** The normal human digestive tract contains about four hundred types of probiotic bacteria that reduce the growth of harmful bacteria and promote a healthy digestive system. Fermented foods are rich in these helpful probiotics. Coconut kefir is no exception and contains large amounts of probiotics. It is also believed to help reduce infections in the digestive tract, prevent (or recover from) diarrhea, and control inflammation.

**ENZYMES:** As a raw food, coconut kefir contains enzymes—proteins that allow certain chemical reactions to take place much faster than they would on their own.

## HEALTH BENEFITS OF COCONUT KEFIR

**INTESTINAL HEALTH:** While no formal studies have been performed on either coconut milk kefir or coconut water kefir, there are numerous studies and abundant anecdotal evidence that promote the health benefits of fermented products such as coconut kefir. Probiotic-rich fermented foods help heal a damaged large intestine, normalize bowel movements, help with digestion, and encourage the body to better assimilate nutrients.

## CHOOSING, USING, AND KEEPING COCONUT KEFIR

The probiotics in kefir are perishable and especially sensitive to warmth. Drink coconut kefir as soon as you open the container or refrigerate it for up to five days (or until the expiration date).

*Caution: Kefir is a healthy beverage as is. There is no need to load it up with sugar! If you do, you'll have converted a healthy food into a sugary soft drink. Resist, resist, resist!!!*

**COCONUT KEFIR IN RECIPES:** Every recipe in this book that uses coconut milk kefir or coconut water kefir was tested using homemade milk kefir, Inner-Eco brand coconut water kefir (1 tablespoon diluted in a cup of water), and Tonix brand coconut water kefir.

**STEPHANIE'S FAVORITE WAY TO USE COCONUT KEFIR:** Coconut water kefir as a summer cooler mixed with fresh-pressed fruit juice and coconut water ice cubes.

# COCONUT NECTAR

Unlike maple syrup, coconut syrup—better known as "nectar"—doesn't come from bark (since coconut palms don't have bark). Coconut syrup is secreted by the coconut palm's blossom stems—largish stems that connect the blossom to the fronds. The same sap is used to make coconut sugar, coconut vinegar, and coconut aminos!

Coconut nectar is considered a raw food—one that is rich in enzymes and amino acids. It contains trace amounts of vitamin C, potassium, phosphorus, magnesium, calcium, zinc, iron, and copper, and also provides small amounts of antioxidant phytonutrients, such as polyphenols, flavonoids, and anthocyanidin.

The mild taste of coconut nectar makes it a favorite with bakers and children, while nutritionists love its low glycemic index ranking of 35. The glycemic index scale measures foods according to the effect they have on blood. It starts at 0 and goes

### VARIETIES OF COCONUT NECTAR

Coconut nectar can vary in color from dark blond to rich brown, depending upon the year's rainfall, time of year when the coconut palm is tapped, and even the heat and fuel source used to reduce the nectar.

to 100. Foods that rate between 0 and 49 have a low glycemic index, foods between 50 and 70 have a moderate glycemic index, and foods that rate over 70 have a high glycemic index. A 2-tablespoon serving of agave nectar, for example, has a glycemic index of 30, placing it in the category of low glycemic foods.

## COCONUT NECTAR: NUTRITION PROFILE PER SERVING (1 TABLESPOON)

**CALORIES:** 55

**AMINO ACIDS:** Coconut nectar contains amino acids, which make up protein in food. When digested, they help the body create solid matter, including skin, eyes, heart, intestines, bones, and muscle. Depending upon which nutrition scientist you ask, there are between twenty and twenty-two amino acids. Of those, eight to ten are considered essential, meaning you must get these from your diet, since your body can't synthesize them from other materials.

**ENZYMES:** As a raw food, coconut nectar is rich in enzymes, the proteins that allow certain chemical reactions to take place much more quickly than those reactions would occur on their own.

**PHOSPHORUS:** Coconut nectar provides trace amounts of phosphorus, a mineral important for bone growth, kidney function, and cell growth.

**POTASSIUM:** Coconut nectar provides trace amounts of potassium, which helps reduce hypertension, regulate blood pressure, and control cholesterol levels and weight.

**CALCIUM:** Coconut nectar provides trace amounts of calcium, a mineral vital for strong bones and teeth, as well as for muscle growth.

**MAGNESIUM:** Coconut nectar provides trace amounts of magnesium, which is essential for metabolism.

**CHLORIDE:** Coconut nectar provides trace amounts of chloride, which corrects the pressure of body fluids and balances the nervous system.

**SULFUR:** Coconut nectar provides trace amounts of sulfur, which is important for healthy hair, skin, and nails, and also helps maintain oxygen balance for proper brain function.

**BORON:** Coconut nectar provides trace amounts of boron, which is essential for healthy bone and joint function, and enhances the body's ability to absorb calcium and magnesium.

**ZINC:** Coconut nectar provides trace amounts of zinc, which is called the "nutrient of intelligence," because it is necessary for mental development.

**MANGANESE:** Coconut nectar provides trace amounts of manganese, which has antioxidant, free-radical-fighting properties. Manganese is important for proper food digestion and normal bone development.

**IRON:** Coconut nectar provides trace amounts of iron, which the body uses to make blood. Iron is necessary for normal mental development in infants and children. It also helps the immune system run efficiently.

**COPPER:** Coconut nectar provides trace amounts of copper, which helps with energy production, as well as melanin production in the skin.

**PHYTOCHEMICALS:** Coconut nectar contains trace amounts of plant chemicals that are powerful antioxidants and help repair and protect cells from free-radical damage. The phytochemicals in coconut nectar include flavonoids (which also have strong anti-inflammatory powers).

## HEALTH BENEFITS OF COCONUT NECTAR

**LOW GLYCEMIC SWEETENER:** Although there have been no formal studies on coconut nectar, its low glycemic status could make it an option, as a sweetener, for individuals with diabetes, prediabetes, and other blood sugar disorders. Anecdotal evidence from coconut-producing countries claims it helps keep the immune system strong, wards off colds and other viral illnesses, and can be used on the skin to treat and prevent breakouts. Talk to your health-care provider about replacing your current sweetener with coconut nectar.

## CHOOSING, USING, AND KEEPING COCONUT NECTAR

Coconut nectar can be kept on a dark shelf in your cupboard for a year or more. (I've kept coconut nectar for two and a half years with no problem.) Look for recipes that have been developed, specifically, with coconut nectar in mind, or find recipes that currently use another liquid sweetener and swap in coconut nectar. Coconut nectar can be used in a 1:1 ratio for honey, maple syrup, brown rice syrup, barley malt, and even agave nectar.

*Caution: Coconut nectar may seem healthier than cane sugar or other liquid sweeteners, but it is still a sweetener. Go easy on it, and remember that your body doesn't need excess sweeteners, no matter what they are made of.*

**COCONUT NECTAR IN RECIPES:** All recipes in this book that use coconut nectar were tested using Coconut Secret brand coconut nectar.

**STEPHANIE'S FAVORITE WAY TO USE COCONUT NECTAR:** My kids love to use it as a syrup over pancakes or as a sweetener for oatmeal and other hot cereals.

# COCONUT SUGAR

Coconut sugar should be considered a "healthier food" rather than a health food per se because, let's face it, no one needs to consume a lot of sweeteners, no matter what they are made of. Coconut sugar is produced by boiling and then dehydrating the sap of the coconut palm. It contains trace amounts of vitamin C, potassium, phosphorus, magnesium, calcium, zinc, iron, and copper, and also supplies small amounts of antioxidant phytonutrients, such as polyphenols, flavonoids, and anthocyanidin.

In 2014, the United Nations' Food and Agriculture Organization named coconut sugar the world's most sustainable sweetener. Coconut palms use minimal amounts of water, especially compared to sugar cane production, and a single coconut palm can continue to produce sap for about twenty years.

Nutritionists love coconut sugar because it ranks low on the glycemic index (a list that measures the effects of carbohydrates on blood sugar). Foods listed high on the glycemic index cause your blood sugar to spike. Fast spikes in blood sugar can also cause your insulin levels to soar in a short period, and this can have serious consequences for diabetics. Coconut sugar ranks just 35 on this index, while regular table sugar (from sugar cane) ranks between 60 and 75.

## COCONUT SUGAR: NUTRITION PROFILE PER SERVING (1 TEASPOON)

**CALORIES:** 20

**PHOSPHORUS:** Coconut sugar provides trace amounts of phosphorus, a mineral important for bone growth, kidney function, and cell growth.

**POTASSIUM:** Coconut sugar provides trace amounts of potassium, which helps reduce hypertension, regulate blood sugar, and control cholesterol levels and weight.

**CALCIUM:** Coconut sugar provides trace amounts of calcium, a mineral vital for strong bones and teeth, as well as muscle growth.

**MAGNESIUM:** Coconut sugar provides trace amounts of magnesium, which is essential for metabolism and nerve health (including helping motor nerves carry messages by electrical impulse between the brain and muscles). Magnesium also stimulates the brain (memory).

**CHLORIDE:** Coconut sugar provides trace amounts of chloride, which corrects the pressure of body fluids, and balances the nervous system.

**SULFUR:** Coconut sugar provides trace amounts of sulfur, which is important for healthy hair, skin, and nails, and also helps maintain oxygen balance for proper brain function.

**BORON:** Coconut sugar provides trace amounts of boron, which is essential for healthy bone and joint function, and enhances the body's ability to absorb calcium and magnesium.

**ZINC:** Coconut sugar provides trace amounts of zinc, which is called the "nutrient of intelligence," because it is necessary for mental development.

**MANGANESE:** Coconut sugar provides trace amounts of manganese, which has antioxidant, free-radical-fighting properties. Manganese is important for proper food digestion and for normal bone growth.

**IRON:** Coconut sugar provides trace amounts of iron, which the body uses to make blood; iron also helps with mental development and the immune system.

**COPPER:** Coconut sugar provides trace amounts of copper, which helps with energy production, as well as melanin production in the skin.

## HEALTH BENEFITS OF COCONUT SUGAR?

**LOW GLYCEMIC SWEETENER:** Although there have been no formal studies on coconut sugar, its low glycemic status could make it an option, as a sweetener, for individuals with diabetes, prediabetes, and other blood sugar disorders. Check with your doctor to see if coconut sugar may be an appropriate sweetener for you.

## CHOOSING, USING, AND KEEPING COCONUT SUGAR

Coconut sugar can be substituted equally for regular (white) cane sugar. Some brands of coconut sugar are especially coarse. If you prefer a finer grain, just process coconut sugar in a coffee grinder or food processor until it comes closer to the consistency of regular cane sugar.

*Caution: In Thailand and other Southeast Asian countries, the term "palm sugar" is commonly used to describe coconut sugar or sugar derived from the sugar palm. Brands that come from these areas may market coconut palm sugar or palm sugar as coconut sugar. When you are shopping, always look for "coconut sugar" on the label (and in the ingredients list).*

**COCONUT SUGAR IN RECIPES:** Regular coconut sugar has been used for the coconut sugar in these recipes.

**STEPHANIE'S FAVORITE WAY TO USE COCONUT SUGAR:** To replace half or all the cane sugar when making baked goods.

---

### BY ANY OTHER NAME . . .

Coconut sugar is also known as coconut crystals, coco sap sugar, coconut palm sugar, and coco sugar.

# COCONUT VINEGAR

Mild-tasting coconut vinegar is made from sap that has been tapped from the thick stem that attaches coconut blossoms to the coconut fronds. This sap, known as "tuba," is then aged for eight months to a year. It is a raw food.

> ### POPULAR IN THE PHILIPPINES
> Coconut vinegar is a staple in Southeast Asia, particularly in the Philippines, where it is called *suka ng niyog*.

## COCONUT VINEGAR: NUTRITION PROFILE PER SERVING (1 TABLESPOON)

**CALORIES:** 0

**POTASSIUM:** While the level of potassium in coconut vinegar hasn't been studied, the same sap used to make the vinegar contains 192 mg per tablespoon. It's thought that coconut vinegar's potassium levels are similar. Potassium is the most important positively charged ion present in the cells of the body. It helps maintain the health of the heart, brain, kidneys, muscle tissues, and other organs of the body. It also plays a key role in the functioning of heart muscle and the contraction of voluntary and involuntary muscles.

**AMINO ACIDS:** Coconut vinegar contains nine essential amino acids, as well as eight nonessential amino acids. For those of you who are not familiar with amino acids, they make up protein in food, and when digested, they help the body create solid matter, including skin, eyes, heart, intestines, bones, and muscle. Depending upon which nutrition scientist you ask, there are between twenty and twenty-two amino acids. Of those, eight to ten are considered essential, meaning you must get these from your diet, as your body can't synthesize them from other materials. Again, this depends upon which nutrition scientist you ask. Some experts believe there are eight essential amino acids, some believe there are nine, and others believe there are ten. Coconut has nine of these that many nutritionists consider essential.

**ENZYMES:** Coconut vinegar is rich in enzymes, the proteins that allow certain chemical reactions to take place much more quickly than those reactions would occur on their own.

**PROBIOTICS:** The normal human digestive tract contains about four hundred types of probiotic bacteria, which reduce the growth of harmful bacteria and promote a healthy digestive system. Fermented foods are rich in these helpful probiotics. Coconut vinegar is no exception, because it contains a large amount of probiotics, and is said to help reduce infections in the digestive tract, prevent (or recover from) diarrhea, and control inflammation.

**PREBIOTICS:** Coconut cider vinegar also contains prebiotics, plant fiber that beneficially nourishes good bacteria that are already present in the large bowel or colon. The body itself does not digest this fiber; instead, the fiber acts as a fertilizer to promote the growth of many of the good bacteria in the gut.

## HEALTH BENEFITS OF COCONUT VINEGAR

**BLOOD SUGAR STABILIZER:** In 2006, a team of researchers out of Arizona State University in Mesa, Arizona, examined the scientific evidence for medicinal uses of coconut and other types of vinegar, focusing particularly on recent investigations supporting vinegar's role as an antiglycemic agent. It was determined that many recent scientific investigations have documented that vinegar does, indeed, stabilize blood sugar. It was also found that vinegar creates a feeling of satiety, which can help with weight control.

## CHOOSING, USING, AND KEEPING COCONUT VINEGAR

Look for a bottle that contains "the mother," a clump of cellulose and other natural material that helps with fermentation.

Coconut vinegar can keep for extended periods if it is stored on a shelf in a dark, cool place. I have a bottle that is two years old and as fresh as it was when I first opened it. Coconut vinegar can be used in any recipe that calls for apple cider vinegar, and it shares the same alkalinizing health benefits (i.e., it helps strengthen the immune system, wards off cravings, and provides quick energy). I enjoy using chilled coconut vinegar as a toner, during the summer, to remove dirt and grime from my skin.

*Caution: Avoid coconut vinegar made from the liquid found in mature coconuts, sometimes called "coconut water vinegar." This "vinegar," a by-product of the coconut oil industry, is made by taking the liquid in brown coconuts and mixing it with a "vinegar starter," and then allowing the mixture to ferment for two to four weeks. It has little nutritional value. You want the traditional vinegar made from the sap of the coconut palm.*

**COCONUT VINEGAR IN RECIPES:** For all recipes that call for coconut vinegar in this book, I use Coconut Secret brand vinegar, which is derived from coconut sap.

**STEPHANIE'S FAVORITE WAY TO USE COCONUT VINEGAR:** Whisked with coconut oil and a bit of salt (and maybe some herbs) as a salad dressing.

# COCONUT AMINOS

Coconut aminos, as a product, is not as well known as coconut oil, coconut milk, coconut water, and coconut flour, so don't worry if you haven't heard of this dark, rich, salty sauce. Made in small batches from the fermented sap of the coconut palm blossoms and mineral-rich sea salt from the Philippines, coconut aminos is used for flavoring, marinating, and dressing food. Think of coconut aminos as soy sauce without the soy.

Small batches ensure that coconut aminos is a raw, enzymatically alive product. It boasts seventeen amino acids and some B vitamins. (Amino acids are the building blocks of proteins in our bodies.) Coconut aminos contains 65 percent less sodium than soy sauce.

Coconut aminos is also a great substitute for Bragg Liquid Aminos, which has the same ingredients as soy sauce, but isn't fermented and contains sixteen amino acids that are not present in soy sauce. If you have issues with soy, you'll have them with Bragg Liquid Aminos.

## COCONUT AMINOS: NUTRITION PROFILE PER SERVING (1 TABLESPOON)

**CALORIES:** 5

**POTASSIUM:** Rich in potassium, coconut aminos has a nearly identical nutrient profile to coconut vinegar. Potassium is the most important positively charged ion present in the cells of the body. It helps maintain the health of the heart, brain, kidneys, muscle tissues, and other organs of the body, and it plays a key role in the contraction of voluntary and involuntary muscles.

**AMINO ACIDS:** Coconut aminos contains nine essential amino acids, as well as eight nonessential amino acids. For those of you who are not familiar with amino acids, they make up protein in food; when digested, they help the body create solid matter, including skin, eyes, heart, intestines, bones, and muscle. Depending upon which nutrition scientist you ask, there are between twenty and twenty-two amino acids. Of those, eight nine or ten are considered essential, meaning you must get these from your diet, as your body can't synthesize them from other materials. Again, this depends upon which nutrition scientist you ask. Some experts believe there are eight essential amino acids, some believe there are nine, and others believe there are ten. Coconut has nine of these that many nutritionists consider essential.

**ENZYMES:** Coconut aminos is rich in enzymes, the proteins that allow certain chemical reactions to take place much more quickly than the reactions would occur on their own.

**PROBIOTICS:** The normal human digestive tract contains about four hundred types of probiotic bacteria, which reduce the growth of harmful bacteria and promote a healthy digestive system. Fermented foods are rich in these helpful probiotics. Coconut aminos is no exception, because it contains large amounts of probiotics, and is said to help reduce infections in the digestive tract, prevent (or recover from) diarrhea, and control inflammation.

## HEALTH BENEFITS OF COCONUT AMINOS

**LARGE INTESTINE HELPER:** Although there have been no formal studies of coconut aminos, anecdotal evidence suggests that this product helps promote a healthy probiotic balance in the large intestine, thanks to its high probiotic content.

## CHOOSING, USING, AND KEEPING COCONUT AMINOS

Coconut aminos is available in glass bottles. If you store it in a dark, cool place, it can keep for a couple of years. Coconut aminos can be used, in a 1:1 ratio, as a substitution for shoyu, tamari-style soy sauces, and Braggs Liquid Aminos (a non-fermented soy product).

*Caution: When choosing coconut aminos, look for products made from the fermented sap of the coconut tree. Avoid products based on coconut water, and ones that have been artificially colored and flavored.*

**COCONUT AMINOS IN RECIPES:** For every recipe in this book that calls for coconut aminos, I've used Coconut Secret, a brand that is derived from coconut sap.

**STEPHANIE'S FAVORITE WAY TO USE COCONUT AMINOS:** As a poultry or pork marinade—whisked with orange juice and flavored with fresh ginger and garlic.

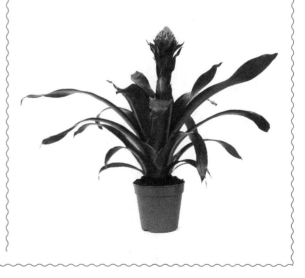

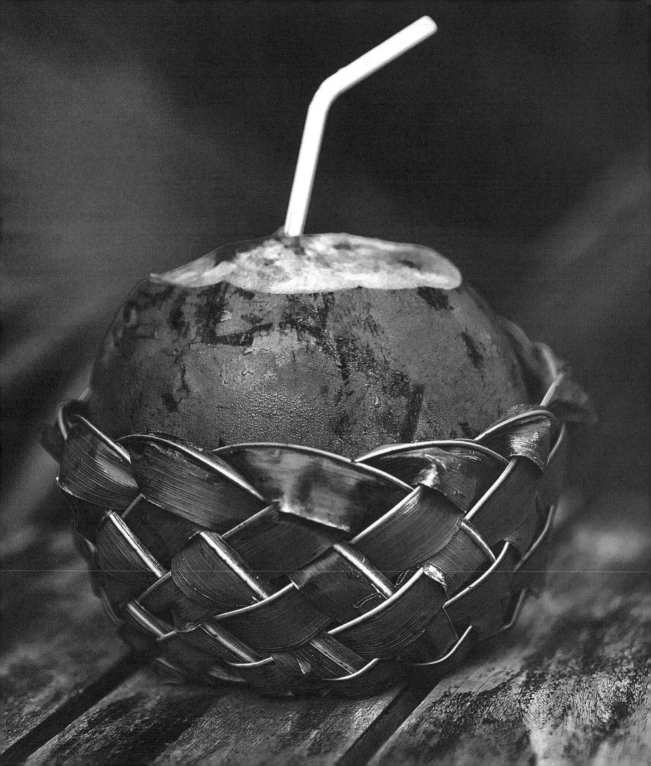

# CHAPTER 3

# DRINK YOUR COCONUT

Mention "coconut," and one of the first things that jumps to mind is coconut water, the almost-clear liquid of young coconuts. With sales increasing by about 42 percent between 2012 and 2013 alone, coconut water is one of today's fastest-growing "health drinks." But coconut water isn't the only coconut beverage to enjoy. Coconut milk—whether homemade, from can, or from a box or carton—is a delicious option for cooking, drinking straight, or making fun flavored drinks like the ones featured here!

You can also use coconut oil, coconut nectar, and coconut crystals to create yummy cocktails, as well as hot and cold drinks that the entire family will enjoy. (Shhh . . . they're also good for you!)

Indeed almost all of coconut's various products lend themselves beautifully to drinks of all kinds, from refreshing electrolyte-filled coconut water–based beverages to creamy blender drinks to hot and frothy coffee house–style treats.

## HOMEMADE COCONUT WATER

*MAKES 1 TO 2 SERVINGS*

While purchasing a Tetra Pack or aseptic box of coconut water is much easier than cracking open a coconut, doing it yourself lets you enjoy an ultra-fresh, clean taste that you just can't get from a packaged product.

So for the intrepid among you, here are instructions for extracting your own coconut water. Have fun!

All you need is 1 young green coconut.

**1.** Place the coconut on an even, sturdy surface. Using your sharpest, heaviest non-serrated knife, cut through the coconut, about 2 or 3 inches from the top, as you would a jack-o'-lantern. Tip: Cutting a square opening instead of a circle will make it easier for you to extract the juice.

**2.** Check the color of the coconut flesh. It should be white. If it is pink or tan or grayish or any other color, it may be going bad.

**3.** Using a spoon, scrape away any flesh that could be in the way of the opening.

**4.** Take a peek at the coconut water (also known as coconut juice; the terms are used interchangeably). It should be clear or slightly milky with no sour smell or taste. If it is an off-color or tastes sour, the coconut water has gone bad.

**5.** Drink the juice straight from the coconut with a straw, or pour it into glasses. Drink immediately, or mix in a squirt of lemon juice to keep the coconut water fresh in your fridge for up to 48 hours. Any unused coconut water can be frozen into ice cubes for use in cooking or for chilling drinks.

**6.** Using a long metal spoon, scoop out the soft flesh. This can be added to smoothies, puddings, blended with fruit and poured into ice pop molds, or eaten straight from the coconut.

## HOMEMADE COCONUT MILK I (MADE WITH A WHOLE COCONUT)

*MAKES 2 TO 4 SERVINGS, DEPENDING UPON THE SIZE OF THE COCONUT*

Making your own coconut milk can be economical and fun, especially if you're looking for an activity to do with your kids that's just a little bit different. And, if you are wary of food or drinks from cans, since some cans are coated with an industrial chemical called bisphenol A (BPA), making your own coconut milk is an easy healthy option.

What many people feel makes BPA harmful is this: It is thought to be an endocrine disrupter, which means it interferes with the production, secretion, and function of natural hormones in a way that is hazardous to your health, possibly leaving individuals susceptible to heart disease, asthma, liver-enzyme abnormalities, type 2 diabetes, reproductive disorders, erectile dysfunction, and breast cancer, as well as reducing the efficacy of chemotherapy treatment.

There's another reason why it's best to stay away from commercially packaged coconut milk: Some brands contain thickeners, gums, or chemical preservatives that your body would be better off without.

1 mature coconut
Room temperature water

**1.** Find the "eyes" of the coconut. Identify the softest eye. Using a corkscrew, pierce the surface and drill into the eye. Once you've burrowed through the shell and reached the interior of the coconut, remove the corkscrew. You can also use the hammer method to find the eye, described in Chapter 2.

**2.** Pour any liquid the mature coconut may contain into a container. Set aside to use in a smoothie. (It is not as fresh-tasting or as nutritious as coconut water from a green coconut, but it is drinkable.)

**3.** For this next step, you'll need a standard screwdriver and hammer. Both clean, please! Position the screwdriver over the top of the coconut, and hit it with the hammer, in order to put a crack in the coconut. Pry open the crack to open the coconut completely into two or more sections.

**4.** Using a spoon, scrape out the white coconut meat. It will be firm. Collect it in a bowl.

**5.** Put a few chunks of coconut meat into a blender. Add water until the coconut is barely covered. Process on the highest power setting until the coconut meat is liquefied, and then pour it into a container.

**6.** Working in batches, continue processing the coconut meat until all of it has been liquefied.

**7.** If you like, pour the blended coconut milk through a fine sieve or cheesecloth to remove any solids. (You can use the solids in baked goods, curries, and smoothies.)

**8.** Store the coconut milk in an airtight container for up to 5 days in the fridge. You can freeze any unused milk in an airtight container for up to 3 months.

# HOMEMADE COCONUT MILK II (MADE WITH DRIED COCONUT)

*MAKES 2 OR MORE 1-CUP SERVINGS*

This is the easy-breezy homemade coconut milk recipe—no coconut opening required! And, because you can choose the amounts of ingredients you want to use, you can also control the amount of coconut milk you can make in one go.

*1  cup or more high-quality, unsweetened shredded dried (also known as shredded or dried) coconut*

*1  cup or more near-boiling water (use 1 cup of water for every cup of dried coconut)*

**1.** Place the unsweetened shredded dried coconut in a blender. Add 1 cup near-boiling water for every cup of coconut you use.

**2.** Process the mixture until it is liquefied, then pour it into a container.

**3.** Allow the coconut milk to cool to room temperature and strain it through a fine sieve or cheesecloth to remove any solids. (You can use the solids in baked goods, curries, and smoothies.)

**4.** Store the coconut milk in an airtight container for up to 5 days in the fridge. You can freeze any unused milk in an airtight container for up to 3 months.

## HOT DRINKS

### MOCHA COCONUT COFFEE

*MAKES ABOUT 3 SERVINGS*

For those of you who love blended, sweet coffee drinks, here is a version that is healthier than the commercial stuff. Yum!

- 1  cup freshly brewed strong coffee (you can use decaf, if desired)
- 1  15-ounce can coconut milk (or 2 cups coconut milk from aseptic box, or refrigerated carton)
- 2  tablespoons organic cocoa powder
- 2  to 3 tablespoons coconut sugar (or sweetener of choice)

  Optional: ¼ teaspoon vanilla extract

**1.** In a medium pot over medium heat, whisk together the coffee and coconut milk.

**2.** Whisk in the cocoa powder. Continue to whisk until no lumps remain.

**3.** Whisk in coconut sugar and, if desired, vanilla. Continue to whisk until sugar has dissolved.

**4.** Remove from heat, and enjoy.

### PUMPKIN COCONUT CHAI LATTE

*MAKES 2 SERVINGS*

I adore pumpkin. I also love how easy it is to sneak into all kinds of foods, from nut butters to baked goods to smoothies to sauces to hot drinks. At one time, pumpkin puree was the only veggie my oldest son would eat. (Well, he wasn't actually aware that he was eating it. . . .) Anyway, you'll love this pumpkin chai!

- ¾  cup water
- 3  chai-flavored tea bags
- ¼  cup pumpkin puree
- 2  cups coconut milk (homemade or from can, aseptic box, or refrigerated carton)
- 1  teaspoon vanilla extract
- ½  to 2 tablespoons coconut sugar (or raw sugar, such as Sucanat)

**1.** Heat water in a medium saucepan until boiling.

**2.** Immediately add tea bags, cover pot, and turn off heat.

**3.** Allow tea bags to steep for 6 minutes.

**4.** Remove tea bags and squeeze all liquid into the pot.

**5.** Turn heat on, to low, and whisk in pumpkin puree, coconut milk, vanilla extract, and sugar, until smooth. Add more water if you want a thinner drink.

- One cup of cubed pumpkin has only 30 calories but 197 percent of an adult's daily requirement of vitamin A.

- Pumpkin also contains vitamins C, B2, B3, B6, and K, as well as manganese, potassium, and magnesium.

- A 1-cup serving of pumpkin contains about 22 percent of an adult's daily requirement of fiber.

- Pumpkin and other winter squash are high in antioxidants and anti-inflammatory compounds that are helpful in cancer prevention and cancer treatment.

- One cup of baked pumpkin (or other winter squash) provides about 340 mg of omega-3 fatty acids in the form of alpha-linolenic acid (ALA).

- Winter squash, such as pumpkin, helps improve blood sugar and insulin regulation, making it an important food for anyone with a blood sugar condition such as prediabetes, hypoglycemia, and type 2 diabetes.

- Pumpkin boasts the ability to block the formation of cholesterol in our cells by inhibiting an enzyme called HMG-CoA reductase. This ability, along with pumpkin's unique antioxidant and anti-inflammatory properties, makes it an important part of a heart-healthy diet.

# COCONUT COCOA

*MAKES 4 SERVINGS*

You'd be much better off health-wise drinking a green drink than hot cocoa. But sometimes life calls for cocoa. When it does, this delicious drink is a much better option than any old dried-chocolate-and-chemical-ridden powdered mix.

- *1 cup canned coconut milk (do not use "lite")*
- *2 cups almond milk or 2 cups additional coconut milk*
- *½ to 1 teaspoon vanilla extract (or a splash of bourbon or rum, for adults)*
- *2 tablespoons organic cocoa powder*
- *4 ounces high-quality raw organic dark chocolate*

**1.** Pour coconut milk, 2 cups almond milk or the additional 2 cups of coconut milk, plus vanilla extract, and cocoa powder into a medium-size pot over low heat.

**2.** Whisk to incorporate.

**3.** As the coconut milk mixture is warming, roughly chop up the dark chocolate.

**4.** Turn the heat up to medium-low and add the chopped dark chocolate. Whisk until melted and combined.

**5.** Remove from heat, and enjoy.

**6.** Leftovers can be stored in the fridge and warmed over low heat.

# COOLERS

## COCONUT COOLER

*MAKES 1 SERVING*

Simple and refreshing—this is everything a cooler should be.

- ¼ *cup coconut milk (homemade or from can, aseptic box, or refrigerated carton)*
- ¼ *cup lime juice*
- 1 *or 2 coconut water ice cubes or regular ice cubes*
- ½ *cup sparkling water*

**1.** In a cocktail shaker, Mason jar, or other type of container with a lid, shake coconut milk and lime juice until well combined.

**2.** Place ice cubes in a glass and pour in coconut milk–lime juice mixture.

**3.** Top off glass with sparkling water.

## HONEYDEW-COCONUT WATER

*MAKES ABOUT 2 SERVINGS*

I adore the soft, sweet, honeysuckle flavor of honeydew. Pairing it with refreshing coconut water makes for a cooling summer drink.

Coconut Simple Syrup:
- 1 *cup water or coconut water*
- ⅓ *cup coconut sugar*

Cooler:
- 4 *cups honeydew melon, cubed (about 2 pounds whole honeydew melon)*
- 1 *cup coconut water*
- 1 *tablespoon coconut simple syrup*
- 1 *to 2 tablespoons fresh lime juice from 1 lime*
- 4 *coconut water ice cubes or regular ice cubes*

**1.** To make the coconut simple syrup, combine water and coconut sugar in a small saucepan. Bring to boil, stirring frequently, then reduce heat and simmer for 10 minutes. Remove from heat and let cool to room temperature. Syrup keeps 2 months in a sealed container in the refrigerator.

**2.** Put the honeydew, coconut water, 1 tablespoon of the simple syrup, and lime juice in a blender and pulse a few times until melon is just broken down into a puree.

**3.** Add the ice cubes and pulse, just until ice is crushed and blended.

NOTE: To easily make ice pops, pour the mixture into ice-pop molds and freeze.

## CITRUS ZINGER

*MAKES 2 SERVINGS*

Refreshing, with the bright tartness of lemons and oranges and the spicy kick of cayenne, this is a real pick-me-up.

*Juice from 3 large juicy lemons*

*Juice from 3 large juicy oranges (preferably juice oranges)*

½  *cup coconut water*

⅛  *teaspoon cayenne pepper*

1  *teaspoon coconut nectar*

**1.** Add all ingredients to a blender. Pulse until cayenne and coconut nectar are distributed.

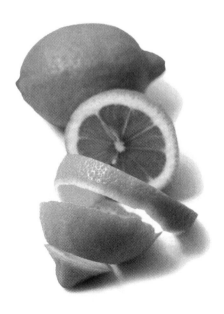

## NATURAL HARD-CORE SPORTS DRINK

*MAKES 4 SERVINGS*

You know all those reports that claim coconut water can be used interchangeably with electrolyte-replacing drinks, such as Gatorade? Well, it's not quite true. While coconut water is an amazingly healthful beverage—and it's great for gentle to moderate exercise (such as walking or an easy softball game)—it doesn't contain the sodium or glucose necessary to replace what's lost during a hard-core, sweaty workout. But if you're someone who loves the idea of a more natural sports drink—one without a neon blue, green, or orange color—I have good news: Coconut water can easily be mixed with a few other ingredients to make the perfect athletic drink.

3½ *cups coconut water (or regular water)*

½  *cup orange juice*

2½ *tablespoons coconut sugar*

¼  *teaspoon salt*

⅛  *teaspoon baking soda*

**1.** Place all ingredients in a blender and process until blended, or add to a covered container and shake until coconut sugar, salt, and baking soda are dissolved and blended.

**2.** Store leftovers in a tightly covered container in the fridge for up to a week.

## SMOOTHIES & OTHER BLENDER DRINKS

## ANOTHER GREEN SMOOTHIE

*MAKES 2 SERVINGS*

I call this "another" green smoothie because the health food world is overflowing with green drink recipes. This one is coconut-based, making it healthful and yummy. Feel free to play with the ingredients. You can replace the banana with mango, omit the fruit, use other greens instead of the spinach, and so on.

- 1 medium ripe banana
- 1 cup fresh (or canned, or frozen) pineapple
- 3 large handfuls fresh spinach (washed)
- 1 cup plain coconut yogurt or coconut kefir
- 6 ounces coconut water (or regular water)
  Optional: 1 tablespoon coconut oil

**1.** Place all ingredients in a blender. Process until smooth.

## BREAKFAST POWER SMOOTHIE

*MAKES 1 TO 2 SERVINGS*

This protein-packed drink is easy for breakfast, but I like it as an afternoon pick-me-up when my energy is dragging. It's so much better for your body than a double latte and chocolate chip cookie!

- 1 cup frozen strawberries (or other berries)
- 1 cup coconut water
- 1 tablespoon creamy roasted almond butter
  Optional: 1 tablespoon coconut sugar
- 1 scoop vegan protein powder of choice (such as brown rice protein powder)
- 1 tablespoon chia seeds
- 3 ice cubes

**1.** Combine berries, coconut water, almond butter, and if desired, coconut sugar in a blender. Process until smooth.

**2.** Blend in protein powder and chia seeds.

**3.** Blend in ice cubes until smooth.

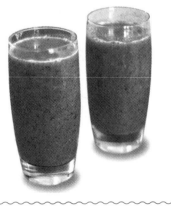

## CANDY BAR SMOOTHIE

*MAKES 2 SERVINGS*

Okay, so there's not really a candy bar in this smoothie, but it sure tastes like one. Try it. Doesn't it remind you of a Mounds or Bounty bar? The difference is, this treat is actually good for you. It's filled with potassium, minerals, and antioxidants.

2   cups coconut milk (homemade or from can, aseptic box, or refrigerated carton)

1   tablespoon coconut oil

¼   cup unsweetened shredded dried coconut

1   tablespoon raw cacao powder

2   pitted Medjool dates

3   to 5 ice cubes

**1.** Place all of the ingredients, except the ice, in a blender and process until completely smooth.

**2.** Add ice cubes and pulse until the mixture is slushy or completely smooth, as desired.

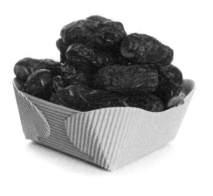

## CHOCO-COCO-MACADAMIA SHAKE

*MAKES 2 SERVINGS*

While it's true that this shake is healthy, it is a rich treat and should probably go into the dessert camp. Enjoy it as a healthful alternative to candy, ice cream, cookies, or other sugary sweets. It is filled with fiber, protein, fatty acids, phytonutrients, vitamins, and minerals—plus chocolate (in the antioxidant-rich form of cacao)!

1½ cups coconut water or coconut milk (homemade or from can, aseptic box, or refrigerated carton)

¼   avocado

1   fresh or frozen banana

10 macadamia nuts

½   cup unsweetened shredded dried coconut
Dash of cinnamon

1   or 2 teaspoons coconut sugar

1   or 2 tablespoons cacao powder or cacao nibs

1   tablespoon coconut oil

**1.** Place all ingredients in a blender. Process until smooth.

## COCO-DREAMSICLE SMOOTHIE

*MAKES 2 SERVINGS*

When I was a kid, Orange Julius drinks were hugely popular. I loved—still love—the orange-vanilla flavor. This updated version features our beloved coconut.

- 2 oranges
- 1 cup unsweetened coconut milk (homemade or from can, aseptic box, or refrigerated carton)
- 1 teaspoon vanilla extract
- 1 tablespoon coconut oil
- 3 to 4 ice cubes

**1.** Segment the oranges (this process is also referred to as "supreming"). To do this, for each orange, slice away the top and bottom. Then take a knife and, starting at the top, slice off the pith and peel. Go all the way around until all of the peel is gone. To remove the orange sections, cut in between the membranes to divide the flesh into its natural segments.

**2.** Put the coconut milk, orange pieces, vanilla, and coconut oil in a blender and process until smooth.

**3.** Add ice and pulse until almost smooth.

## NUTTY ORANGE SHAKE

*MAKES 2 SERVINGS*

This shake is loaded with beta-carotene and fiber from carrots and papaya (or mango). The citrus juices add potassium and vitamin C, and the nuts add protein. This is a terrific way for those veggie-phobes in your life to get their produce.

- ¼ cup chopped pistachios, almonds, or skinless hazelnuts
- 1 cup diced ripe papaya or mango
- 1 small carrot, peeled and chopped
- ⅔ cup freshly squeezed orange juice
- 1 cup coconut milk (homemade or from can, aseptic box, or refrigerated carton)
- 1 tablespoon lime juice
- 2 teaspoons coconut sugar
- 3 or 4 ice cubes

**1.** Place all of the ingredients, except the ice, in a blender and process at high speed until completely smooth.

**2.** Add ice cubes and pulse until the mixture is slushy or completely smooth, as desired.

## COCO-PECAN SHAKE

*MAKES 2 SERVINGS*

Ooh . . . this is luscious. And protein-filled. It also has plenty of fiber. And did I mention how nutty and delicious it is?

- 1 cup coconut water
- 1 cup coconut milk (homemade or from can, aseptic box, or refrigerated carton)
- ½ cup pecan pieces
- 1 tablespoon chia seeds
- 1 banana or small, ripe peeled pear
- 1 teaspoon coconut nectar
- 1 teaspoon pure vanilla extract
  Pinch of sea salt

**1.** Place all ingredients in a blender. Process until smooth.

## COCO PINEAPPLE PEPITA SMOOTHIE

*MAKES 2 SERVINGS*

This is another wonderfully unique, healthful smoothie, packed with protein, minerals, antioxidants, omega-3 fatty acids, and all the health benefits of coconut. It truly is a meal (or, at the very least, a hearty snack) in a glass.

- 2 cups fresh or frozen pineapple chunks
- ½ cup freshly squeezed orange juice
- 2 tablespoons raw pepitas (green, hulled pumpkin seeds)

- 1 slice ginger, peeled
- 1 teaspoon coconut sugar
- 1 tablespoon fresh lime juice
- 1 cup coconut milk (homemade or from can, aseptic box, or refrigerated carton)
- 3 or 4 ice cubes

**1.** Place all of the ingredients, except the ice, in a blender and process at high speed until completely smooth.

**2.** Add ice cubes and pulse until the mixture is slushy or completely smooth, as desired.

## CREAMY AVOCADO SHAKE

*MAKES 2 SERVINGS*

This shake is creamy and dairy-like, making it ideal for anyone who is trying to cut out dairy, but who misses the silkiness of milk.

- ½ avocado
- ½ cup coconut milk (homemade or from can, aseptic box, or refrigerated carton)
- ½ cup coconut water
- ¼ cup plain coconut yogurt or kefir
- ½ fresh or frozen banana
- 2 tablespoons coconut butter or dried unsweetened coconut
- 2 ice cubes

*Optional: ½ teaspoon vanilla extract*

**1.** Place all ingredients in a blender. Process until smooth.

## GREEN COCONUT VANILLA NUT SMOOTHIE

*MAKES 2 SERVINGS*

You just can't go wrong combining macadamia nuts and coconut! This smoothie is filled with healthy fat. Plus, it's a great way to use the pulp from all those green coconuts you may be cracking open for their water!

- 1   *cup coconut water*
- ½   *cup packed young coconut pulp (or ¼ cup unsweetened shredded dried coconut)*
- ⅓   *cup macadamia nuts*
- ½   *teaspoon pure vanilla extract*
- ½   *tablespoon coconut nectar*

**1.** Place all ingredients in a blender and process until smooth and creamy.

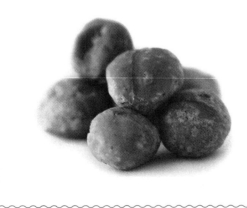

## KEY LIME–COCONUT FRAPPE

*MAKES 2 SERVINGS*

All three of my sons and I have January birthdays. Because we each enjoy key lime pie on our special days, January is dubbed "Lime Pie Month" in our household. Is it any wonder that this is one of our favorite blender drinks?

- 1   *cup coconut milk (homemade or from can, aseptic box, or refrigerated carton)*
- ¼   *teaspoon grated lime rind*
     *Juice from 1 lime or two key limes*
- 1   *tablespoon coconut nectar or sugar*
- 1   *tablespoon coconut oil*
- ¼   *cup unsweetened shredded dried coconut*
- 3   *ice cubes*

**1.** Place first 6 ingredients in a blender; process until smooth.

**2.** Add ice cubes and pulse until smooth.

## OUTRAGEOUS MORNING SMOOTHIE

*MAKES 2 SERVINGS*

This superfood-packed smoothie is a great way to give your body a lot of good stuff at once. Have one of these for breakfast and you'll be able to work well past lunchtime without snacking! You'll need a powerful blender for this one.

- 1 *large handful roughly chopped kale, spinach, or collards, or a combination of these greens*
- 1 *cup frozen mango chunks*
- 1 *cup coconut water*
- 2 *tablespoons almond butter*
- 1 *tablespoon chia seeds*
  *Optional: squirt of lemon or lime*

**1.** Place all ingredients in a blender and process until completely uniform in color and all the bits of green are pulverized. Serve immediately.

## TROPICAL FRUIT SLUSHY

*MAKES 2 SERVINGS*

I prefer this tangy smoothie as an afternoon treat or even a dessert. Once you've tried it, it will become a favorite!

- 1 *cup fresh or frozen pineapple chunks (or a combination of pineapple and mango chunks)*
- 1 *cup coconut milk (homemade or from can, aseptic box, or refrigerated carton)*
- 1 *teaspoon finely chopped ginger*
- 3 *or 4 ice cubes*

**1.** Place the first 3 ingredients in a blender and process until smooth.

**2.** Add ice cubes and blend on high speed until slushy.

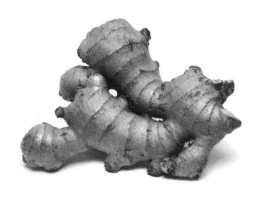

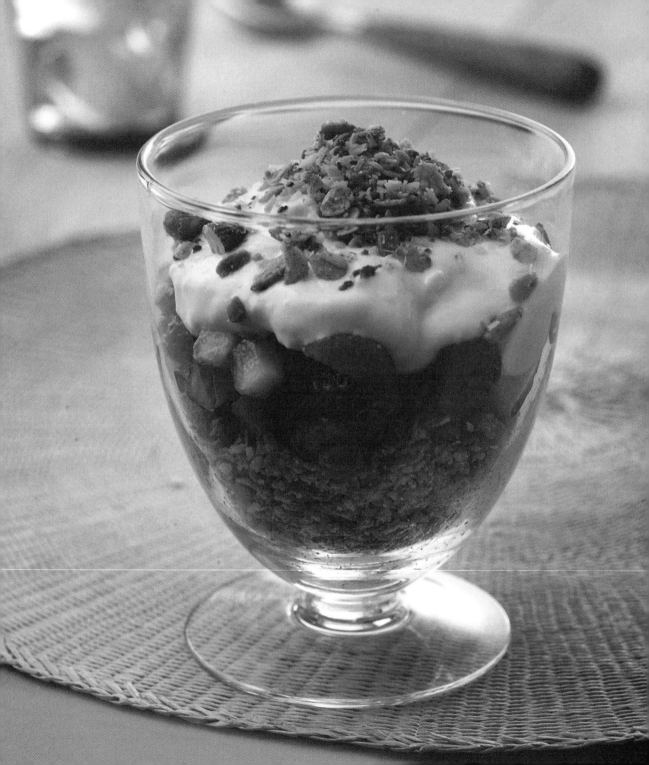

# CHAPTER 4

# BREAKFAST: START YOUR DAY WITH COCONUT

Coconut is a natural breakfast food. It marries so well—in all of its forms—with so many of the foods typically enjoyed in the morning. Plus, it provides a range of nutrients that help start the day powerfully. The antioxidant levels in coconut help slow or stop damage to healthy tissues, as well as strengthen the immune system. Coconut also has protein for sustained energy, fiber for a feeling of fullness and steady blood sugar levels, and healthy fats to keep your brain running efficiently and your heart healthy. In this chapter, I share some of my favorite ways to enjoy coconut for breakfast. If you want to start your day off even more healthily, enjoy a green drink with breakfast, as I do. (Check out Chapter 3 for great coconut-based beverages.)

## CEREAL HOT & COLD

### COCONUT PORRIDGE

*MAKES 1 SERVING*

Based on coconut, high-protein nuts, and chia, this porridge is a favorite of Paleo eaters, who appreciate its omega-3 fatty acids, fiber, and other nutrients. You can dress up this cereal—hot or cold—with chopped nuts, seeds, or fruit. If you want a thicker porridge, just add a little more chia.

*²⁄₃ cup coconut milk (homemade or from can, aseptic box, or refrigerated carton)*

*1 tablespoon chia seeds*

*¼ cup unsweetened shredded dried coconut*
*Pinch of salt*

*2 tablespoons almond meal (or ground cashews, walnuts, pecans, or other nuts)*

*1 tablespoon coconut sugar or nectar, or to taste*

*Optional: splash of vanilla or almond extract*

**1.** In a small saucepan, over medium-low heat, add milk and whisk in chia seeds. Cook for 1 or 2 minutes.

**2.** Whisk in remaining ingredients and turn heat to medium-high. Cook until porridge reaches desired thickness.

OPPOSITE: **Coconut Granola, page 64**

# COCONUT GRANOLA

*MAKES 5 CUPS*

Coconut granola is not super sweet, but it is dense in protein, fiber, omega-3 fatty acids, heart-and-brain-healthy fats, and antioxidants, making it a great way to start the day, especially if you enjoy it with fresh fruit. Berries are particularly nice—and don't forget the coconut yogurt if you want to make a pretty breakfast parfait that tastes like dessert.

**NOTE:** A serving is about ⅓ cup, although most people (including me) tend to eat much more at one sitting.

> *Coconut oil for greasing the pan*
> *¼ cup nut butter (almond, peanut, cashew, sunflower, or other nut)*
> *⅓ cup coconut oil, melted*
> *⅓ to ½ cup coconut sugar*
> *½ teaspoon salt*
> *½ teaspoon cinnamon*
> *2½ cups old-fashioned or steel-cut oats*
> *1½ cups quinoa flakes (or an additional cup of oats)*
> *1 cup unsweetened shredded dried coconut*
> *¼ cup chia seeds*
> *1 cup almonds, or other nuts, chopped*
> *1 cup sunflower seeds (or other nuts or seeds, chopped)*

**1.** Preheat oven to 300°F.

**2.** Lightly grease 2 or 3 baking sheets with a very small amount of coconut oil.

**3.** In a large saucepan over medium heat, whisk together the nut butter, coconut oil, coconut sugar, salt, and cinnamon until mixture is combined and smooth.

**4.** Turn off heat and stir in oats, quinoa flakes, shredded coconut, and chia seeds, completely coating oats in the nut butter–coconut oil mixture.

**5.** Stir in almonds and sunflower seeds until coated.

**6.** Scrape mixture onto cookie sheets in a thin, single layer, being careful not to crowd granola on top of each other. (Note: If you like chunky granola like I do, pinch pieces together into chunks.)

**7.** Place baking sheet on middle shelf of oven and bake for 10 minutes.

**8.** Stir and bake for another 8 to 10 minutes until granola is golden brown. Do not overbake granola—it will continue to cook after you remove it from the oven, so you want it to be a bit sticky when you take it out.

**9.** Allow granola to completely cool and firm up (about an hour) before eating or storing in airtight canisters in a cool, dry place.

**10.** For a pretty presentation, serve the granola layered with coconut yogurt and fresh berries.

# BAKED BANANA OATMEAL

*MAKES 4 SERVINGS*

Baked oatmeal is a fun make-ahead dish for brunch and great for feeding a crowd (go ahead and double the recipe, if you're so inclined). This version is especially delicious and especially nutritious, thanks to the vitamins from the fruit, protein from the walnuts, and all the goodies that coconut provides. But feel free to play: Use a different nut. Experiment with different fruit. Throw in a handful of raisins. Add more sweetener. Try almond extract in place of the vanilla. You get the picture.

*Coconut oil for greasing the pan*

2  *cups chopped fresh fruit of choice (such as bananas, apples, or peaches)*

2  *cups old-fashioned or steel-cut oats (not instant)*

1  *teaspoon cinnamon*

½  *teaspoon allspice*

½  *teaspoon salt*

1  *teaspoon baking powder*

½  *cup chopped walnuts*

1  *egg*

2  *cups coconut milk (homemade or from can, aseptic box, or refrigerated carton)*

¼  *cup coconut nectar*

1  *teaspoon vanilla*

2  *tablespoons unsweetened shredded dried coconut*

**1.** Preheat oven to 375°F.

**2.** Grease an 8-by-8-inch baking dish with coconut oil.

**3.** Evenly layer the bottom of the baking dish with fruit.

**4.** In a medium bowl, whisk together oats with cinnamon, allspice, salt, baking powder, and chopped walnuts.

**5.** In a separate bowl, whisk together the egg, coconut milk, coconut nectar, and vanilla.

**6.** Spoon oat mixture over the fruit.

**7.** Carefully pour the liquid mixture over the oats. Gently tilt the pan to ensure liquid evenly covers dry ingredients.

**8.** Scatter shredded coconut across the top.

**9.** Bake for 40 minutes or until the top is golden and the oatmeal is firm to the touch.

**10.** Allow to cool slightly before slicing.

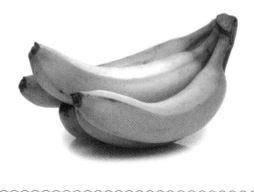

## CREAMY MILLET PORRIDGE

*MAKES 2 SERVINGS*

I love millet, a seed that is high in minerals, fiber, protein, and antioxidants. This recipe is a fun, different take on hot cereal, with millet playing the leading role.

⅔ cup uncooked millet

1 tablespoon unrefined coconut oil

1½ cups unsweetened coconut milk
   (homemade or from can, aseptic box,
   or refrigerated carton)

1 cup coconut water or plain water,
   preferably at room temperature

½ cup chopped nuts or sunflower seeds

Sweetener of choice

**1.** Place millet in a food processor, blender, or even a clean coffee grinder and pulse 2 or 3 times until the millet is coarsely ground. Don't overdo this—you don't want flour!

**2.** Warm coconut oil in a small saucepan over medium heat.

**3.** Add pulsed millet to the saucepan and sauté for 2 to 4 minutes, or until lightly toasted.

**4.** Slowly add coconut milk and water, and stir.

**5.** Bring millet to a gentle simmer and, stirring occasionally, cook until mixture is porridge-like.

**6.** Ladle into serving bowls and top with chopped nuts and sweetener.

### EASY "COCONUTTY" PORRIDGE

Do you want to know the easiest way to add coconut to your hot cereal? Simply replace water with an equal measure of coconut milk or coconut water, and substitute butter or the oil you usually use with coconut oil or coconut butter. If you use sweetener, switch to coconut sugar or nectar. And for a fun texture, add a flurry of shredded coconut. Easy-peasy!

## TOASTED COCONUT AMARANTH PORRIDGE

*MAKES 2 SERVINGS*

Are you familiar with amaranth? It's a Mexican seed that contains 26 g of protein and 13 g of fiber per cup! The same amount also provides large percentages of the daily recommended allowances of magnesium (119 percent), iron (81 percent), vitamin B6 (55 percent), and calcium (30 percent). There is a downside to amaranth, though: It is slightly bitter—but can easily be made tasty with a little coconut! This recipe passes the picky kid test with flying colors.

1½ cups water

½ cup uncooked amaranth
   Pinch of salt

1 teaspoon coconut oil

½ cup coconut milk (homemade or from can,
   aseptic box, or refrigerated carton)

¼ *cup unsweetened shredded dried coconut*

¼ *cup chopped walnuts, pecans, or almonds*

  *Optional: coconut sugar, coconut nectar, or other sweetener, to taste*

**1.** In a small saucepan with a tight-fitting lid, bring water to a boil. Add the amaranth and salt, reduce heat, and cover, simmering for 20 minutes, or until the water is absorbed.

**2.** Remove from heat and stir in the coconut oil, coconut milk, shredded coconut and chopped nuts.

**3.** Serve immediately with optional sweetener.

## BERRY GOOD!
### RED BERRY SAUCE
*MAKES ABOUT 1 CUP*

Looking for something yummy to spoon on your oatmeal, pancakes, or anything else? Enjoy this fresh-tasting recipe for homemade sauce.

1½ *cups frozen strawberries, raspberries, or a mix*

3  *tablespoons coconut nectar*

  *Squirt of lemon or lime juice*

1½ *tablespoons chia seeds*

**1.** In a medium saucepan over medium heat, combine the frozen berries and coconut nectar. Cover and simmer, stirring frequently.

**2.** Cook about 5 minutes, or until berries are soft and beginning to break down.

**3.** Remove from heat and add lemon juice.

**4.** Lightly mash the berries with a fork or potato masher to desired chunkiness.

**5.** Stir in chia seeds and transfer mixture to an airtight container. Allow to firm up in refrigerator 3 hours or overnight before using.

# DECADENT BREAKFAST QUINOA

*MAKES 2 SERVINGS*

Oh, quinoa! How I do love thee! I love your 24 g of protein and 12 g of fiber per cup. I love your high mineral content. I love that you contain nine of the essential amino acids (which cannot be made by the body and therefore must come from food), thereby making you a complete protein. I love your delicate crunch and your versatility and how energized I feel after I eat you. And I love you in this yummy breakfast recipe. Yes I do.

> *Coconut oil for greasing pan*
>
> ½  *cup water*
>
> ½  *cup canned coconut milk*
>
> 2   *tablespoons sweet potato or pumpkin puree*
>
> ¼  *cup uncooked quinoa*
>
> 1   *tablespoon coconut nectar or maple syrup*
>
> 2   *teaspoons coconut oil*
>
> ¼  *teaspoon vanilla extract*
>
> ½  *teaspoon ground cinnamon*
>
> ¼  *teaspoon ground ginger*
>
> ¼  *teaspoon allspice*
>
> 1   *tablespoon coconut oil, melted*
>
> 1   *tablespoon maple syrup*
>
> 1½ *tablespoons finely ground almond flour*
>
> ¼  *cup pecans, chopped*

## WHY QUINOA NEEDS TO BE RINSED BEFORE COOKING

Rinsing removes saponin, which is quinoa's natural coating. This coating can have a bitter or soapy taste. The easiest way to remove it is to dump the uncooked quinoa into a fine-mesh strainer and let cold water run over it for a minute or two. Allow the grain to drip-dry and continue with your recipe. If you don't have a fine-mesh strainer, try the following: Place uncooked quinoa in the bottom of a large mixing bowl, cover it with cold water—by an inch or two—and then give the mix a vigorous stir. Allow the bowl of quinoa and water to sit untouched while you do the laundry, make phone calls, or help a kid with his or her piano practice or homework (maybe about 10 minutes or more, if you'd like). Then come back, pour off the water, dump the soggy quinoa into a skillet, and let the excess water cook off over low heat. Then continue with the recipe.

**1.** Preheat oven to 350°F.

**2.** Lightly grease a small (4-cup) casserole dish or baking dish.

**3.** In a small bowl, whisk together water, coconut milk, pumpkin, quinoa, maple syrup, 2 teaspoons coconut oil, vanilla, cinnamon, ginger, and allspice, until thoroughly combined. Pour into prepared dish.

**4.** Cover with foil or lid and bake for 45 minutes.

**5.** While the quinoa bakes, make topping: Add the melted coconut oil, maple syrup, almond flour, and pecans to a bowl. Stir to combine.

**6.** Remove baked quinoa from oven, take off cover, sprinkle with topping, and return to oven, uncovered, to bake for another 10 minutes, or until browned.

**7.** Allow to cool slightly before serving.

## FROM THE GRIDDLE

### COCONUT FLOUR PANCAKES

*MAKES 2 SERVINGS*

This no-grain pancake is a Paleo favorite. You won't feel sluggish or bloated after eating these beauties! These protein-rich pancakes make for a fun weekend breakfast when paired with veggie juice and maybe a salad or some fruit.

*4   eggs*

*1   cup coconut milk (homemade or from can, aseptic box, or refrigerated carton)*

*1   tablespoon coconut water or plain water (more if batter looks too thick)*

*1   teaspoon vanilla extract*

*1   tablespoon coconut nectar*

*½   cup coconut flour*

*1   teaspoon baking soda*

*¼   teaspoon salt*

*2   tablespoons unsweetened shredded dried coconut*

*1   or 2 teaspoons coconut oil for the skillet*

**1.** In a small bowl, beat eggs until frothy.

**2.** Mix in coconut milk, water, vanilla, and coconut nectar. Set aside.

**3.** In a large bowl, whisk together coconut flour, baking soda, and salt until thoroughly combined and no lumps remain. Stir in shredded coconut.

**4.** Add egg–coconut milk mixture to dry ingredients and stir until well blended.

**5.** Add a teaspoon of coconut oil to a skillet over medium heat. Ladle in about 2 tablespoons of batter per pancake, spreading a bit with the back of a spoon if necessary.

**6.** Cook 2 or 3 minutes on each side, or until pancake begins to brown.

**7.** Serve immediately with your favorite toppings.

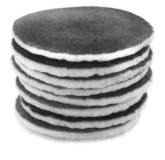

# COCONUT WAFFLES

*MAKES 3 SERVINGS*

These showcase coconut in four forms to help improve the health of your brain, heart, and immune system.

- ⅓ cup sweetened or unsweetened dried shredded coconut
- 4 tablespoons coconut oil
- 6 large eggs
- 3 tablespoons coconut nectar
- 1 teaspoon vanilla extract
- 2 tablespoons pumpkin, sweet potato, banana, apple, or pear puree
- ⅓ cup coconut flour
- ¼ teaspoon salt
- ½ teaspoon cinnamon
- ½ teaspoon baking soda

**1.** Place a rack in the center of the oven and preheat to 350°F.

**2.** Place coconut on a baking sheet and toast in the oven for about 4 minutes. Keep an eye on the coconut, as it browns and burns quickly.

**3.** Remove toasted coconut from the oven and set aside.

**4.** In a medium bowl, whisk together coconut oil, eggs, coconut nectar, vanilla extract, and the puree. Whisk until well incorporated.

**5.** In a small bowl, whisk together the coconut flour, salt, cinnamon, and baking soda. Continue whisking until all lumps are gone.

**6.** Whisk the dry ingredients from the small bowl into the wet ingredients.

**7.** Stir in the toasted, shredded coconut. Allow mixture to sit for 5 minutes while you plug in and preheat the waffle iron.

**8.** Bake waffles according to the manufacturer's directions for using your waffle iron.

**9.** To keep finished waffles from getting cold, cover and keep them in a warm oven until serving time.

**10.** Freeze leftovers and reheat them in a toaster.

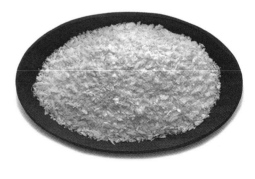

# TROPICAL TOPPER
## PINEAPPLE COCONUT SYRUP

*MAKES 3½ CUPS*

1   cup coconut water or plain water
½   cup coconut sugar
3   cups chopped fresh or frozen pineapple
    Squirt of lemon or lime juice

**1.** Whisk together the first 3 ingredients in a saucepan over medium heat.

**2.** Bring to a boil. Let boil for 5 to 7 minutes until liquid has been reduced and pineapple is soft.

**3.** Puree ingredients with a squirt of lemon juice in a blender until smooth.

**4.** Use immediately or let the syrup cool and then store in an airtight container in the refrigerator.

## COCONUT SYRUP

*MAKES 1½ CUPS*

1   15-ounce can coconut milk
½   cup coconut sugar
    Dash of vanilla or almond extract or lemon juice

**1.** Whisk together all ingredients in a saucepan over medium heat.

**2.** Cook, stirring constantly, just until mixture comes to a boil.

**3.** Quickly reduce the heat to medium and let simmer for 15 to 20 minutes until mixture thickens into a syrup, being very, very careful not to let it cook at a full boil.

**4.** Use immediately or let the syrup cool and then store in an airtight container in the refrigerator.

## COCONUT FRENCH TOAST

*MAKES 6 SERVINGS*

The nutritionist in me encourages you to pair this sweet, rich dish with a green drink and maybe a side of protein.

- 4 *large eggs*
- 2 *tablespoons coconut nectar*
- ½ *cup coconut milk (homemade or from can, aseptic box, or refrigerated carton)*
- ¼ *cup orange juice*
- 4 *to 6 slices whole grain, gluten-free, spelt, or wheat bread*
- 1 *to 2 tablespoons coconut oil*
  *Optional toppings, including coconut nectar, applesauce, maple syrup, fruit, nut butter, etc.*

**1.** Whisk together the eggs, coconut nectar, coconut milk, and orange juice in a shallow pan or baking dish until well blended.

**2.** Add the bread slices and let them soak in the mixture for 1 minute on each side, or until bread is saturated.

**3.** Heat coconut oil in one or two griddles or frying pans over medium heat.

**4.** Add bread slices, cooking for 2 or 3 minutes per side, or until golden and crispy.

**5.** Serve with optional toppings, as desired.

## EGGS

## QUICHE

*MAKES 6 SERVINGS*

Quiche is a fantastic make-ahead, feed-a-crowd dish for breakfast, brunch, lunch, or even dinner. Instead of all the fatty, artery-clogging heavy cream and cheese so many quiches contain, this one relies on coconut for its rich, creamy texture. This is yet another recipe you can play with and customize to suit your own taste. Please experiment with the veggies, herbs, spices, and even the crust (or be bold and try it without the crust!).

- 1 *cup canned coconut milk (do not use "lite")*
- 4 *large eggs*
- 1 *teaspoon dry mustard powder*
- 1 *tablespoon liquid coconut oil*
- 3 *cups chopped vegetables (leeks, sweet bell peppers, zucchini, asparagus, mushrooms, broccoli, spinach, kale, etc.)*
- ¼ *teaspoon salt*
- ¼ *teaspoon pepper*
- 1 *8- or 9-inch whole grain, regular, or gluten-free piecrust, unbaked and in a pie pan*
- 1 *tablespoon minced chives, tarragon, minced green onion tops, or parsley*

1. Preheat oven to 350°F.

2. Whisk together coconut milk, eggs, and mustard powder. Set aside.

3. Add coconut oil to a large skillet. Sauté vegetables over medium heat until just softened, about 3 to 5 minutes. (Or simply open the fridge and pull out 3 cups of cooked veggies from last night's dinner.) Season with salt and pepper.

4. Put sautéed vegetables into unbaked piecrust. Add egg mixture and sprinkle with chives and tarragon.

5. Bake quiche for 45 minutes or until done. A knife inserted in center of filling should come out clean.

## FRITTATA

*MAKES 4 SERVINGS*

Frittatas are a great make-ahead option for egg lovers who want an easy way to sneak more veggies into their diet. Play around with this recipe—try spinach or another green instead of the kale, or throw in a sautéed zucchini or last night's chopped vegetables. Use a shallot instead of the onion. But keep the coconut! You want all of its heart-healthy and brain-boosting benefits!

8 *large eggs*

½ *cup canned coconut milk*

    *Salt and pepper, to taste*

1 *tablespoon coconut oil*

⅓ *cup chopped onion*

½ *cup chopped red pepper*

2 *cups chopped baby kale*

1. Preheat oven to 350°F.

2. In a medium bowl, whisk together the eggs and coconut milk. Add salt and pepper. Set aside.

3. In a medium-size ovenproof skillet, heat coconut oil over medium heat. Add onion and red pepper and sauté for 3 minutes, until onion is translucent.

4. Add kale and cook until it wilts, about 3 minutes.

5. Add eggs to vegetables in the skillet. Cook for about 4 minutes until the bottom and edges of the frittata start to set.

6. Put frittata in the oven and cook for about 10 minutes, until the frittata is cooked all the way through.

7. Slice and serve.

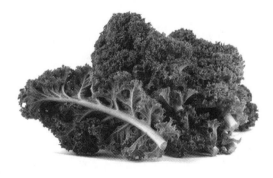

## OMELET

*MAKES 1 OR 2 SERVINGS*

From a health standpoint, omelets are a great way to gussy up any blend of veggies—just use them as a filling! Here, coconut lends healthful lauric acid and medium chain fatty acids to the mix. You provide the herbs and veggies.

3  *large eggs*

⅔  *cup canned coconut milk*

¼  *cup chopped cooked vegetables of choice (this is a great way to deliciously use up last night's leftover veggie sauté)*

1  *to 3 tablespoons herbs of choice*

   *Optional: ½ tablespoon unsweetened shredded dried coconut*

   *Salt and pepper, to taste*

2  *teaspoons coconut oil*

**1.** Whisk eggs together in a bowl and add coconut milk, veggies, herbs, optional shredded coconut, salt, and black pepper.

**2.** Warm coconut oil in small skillet over medium heat. When warm, pour in egg mixture and swirl to coat the bottom of the pan. Stir once or twice and then stop! You want to allow the omelet to set.

**3.** Flip after cooking omelet 2 to 3 minutes and cook for another minute or two until eggs are cooked all the way through.

## SUPER EASY BREAKFAST CASSEROLE

*MAKES 8 SERVINGS*

This easy make-ahead meal is a great way to slip a bit of coconut into your day, so think about it for your next brunch. I wouldn't make it your entire meal, though—I suggest adding a green salad or a veggie juice.

1  *tablespoon liquid coconut oil*

10 *slices of whole grain bread (regular or gluten-free) or leftover rolls*

1  *cup chopped banana, apple, pear, berries, or other fruit*

¼  *cup unsweetened shredded dried coconut*

3  *cups coconut milk (homemade or from can, aseptic box, or refrigerated carton)*

7  *eggs*

1  *to 2 teaspoons vanilla*

**1.** Preheat oven to 350°F.

**2.** Lightly grease a 9-by-13-inch baking dish with a bit of the coconut oil and set aside the remaining oil to use in the recipe.

**3.** Tear the bread into bite-size pieces and arrange evenly in the bottom of the baking dish.

**4.** Scatter the fruit, distributing it evenly over the bread.

**5.** Sprinkle the shredded coconut, distributing it evenly, over the fruit.

**6.** In a medium bowl, whisk together the coconut milk, eggs, vanilla, and reserved coconut oil until thoroughly combined. Pour the milk mixture over the ingredients in the baking dish, covering all pieces.

**7.** Bake for 35 to 40 minutes, keeping an eye on the top of the casserole. Cover it with foil if it starts to burn.

**8.** Remove casserole from oven when puffy and firm.

**9.** Allow to cool for 15 minutes before serving.

## BREAKFAST BAKED GOODS

## OATMEAL BANANA BREAKFAST BARS

*MAKES 9 BARS*

If you love bars, do something nice for yourself and your family: Make your own. This coconut-rich version is a great starter recipe.

Coconut oil for greasing the pan

2 cups old-fashioned oats (or 1 cup oats and 1 cup flaked quinoa)

1 cup unsweetened shredded dried coconut

¼ cup chia seeds

½ cup chopped walnuts, pecans, almonds, or other nuts

½ cup finely chopped dried fruit (apricots, peaches, tart cherries, etc.)

½ cup sunflower seeds

½ teaspoon salt

¾ cup mashed banana (or very thick applesauce or pear sauce)

1 egg

½ cup coconut sugar

3 tablespoons liquid coconut oil

Splash of vanilla or almond extract

**1.** Preheat oven to 375°F.

**2.** Grease an 8-inch square baking pan.

**3.** In a large bowl, stir together oats, shredded coconut, chia, walnuts, dried fruit, sunflower seeds, and salt. Set aside.

**4.** In a medium bowl, mix together mashed banana, egg, coconut sugar, coconut oil, and either vanilla or almond extract until smooth and thoroughly combined.

**5.** Add banana mixture to oats and stir until evenly incorporated.

**6.** Scrape mixture into prepared pan and smooth the surface.

**7.** Bake until bars are golden brown, about 25 minutes.

**8.** Allow to cool before cutting into 9 bars.

# SIMPLE COCONUT FLOUR MUFFINS

*MAKES ABOUT 12 STANDARD MUFFINS OR 24 MINI MUFFINS*

This is a grain-free muffin recipe. It is an awesome way to pack protein, fiber, and the healing benefits of coconut into a tasty package. That said, baking with coconut flour is a bit different than baking with wheat-based flour or even a gluten-free all-purpose flour. For one thing, coconut flour typically needs a lot of eggs to create the finished product, which might be a little denser than you're used to. But this recipe yields a delicious muffin—and it's versatile, too: Feel free to experiment with the sweetener, add different nuts or seeds (even a tablespoon of chia!), or introduce a ½ cup of dried fruit or chopped fresh fruit and whatever spices you'd like. Balance this with some veggie juice and a side of protein and your day is off to a great start!

- ¾  cup coconut flour

    Optional: ¼ cup unsweetened shredded dried coconut

- ½  teaspoon baking soda

    Large pinch of salt

- 6  eggs

- ½  cup liquid coconut oil

- ½  cup coconut nectar

- ½  to 1 teaspoon vanilla or almond extract, or a dash of cinnamon

**1.** Preheat oven to 350°F.

**2.** In a small bowl, whisk together coconut flour, optional shredded coconut, baking soda, and salt. Set aside.

**3.** In a medium bowl, whisk together eggs, coconut oil, coconut nectar, and vanilla.

**4.** Add liquid ingredients to the dry ingredients and mix until thoroughly combined. Allow batter to sit for 5 minutes (this allows the coconut flour and shredded coconut to absorb the liquid fully) while you prepare the muffin tins.

**5.** Prepare 12 standard or 24 mini-muffin cups by lightly greasing with coconut oil or lining with paper muffin liners.

**6.** Scrape batter into prepared muffin pan, filling each cup about ⅔ of the way.

**7.** Bake for about 25 minutes, or until muffins become golden and are firm to the touch.

**8.** Allow muffins to cool for 15 minutes before removing from them from pan.

# BRUNCH CAKE

*SERVES 12*

Try as I might, I can't condone eating cake for breakfast—at least not on a regular basis. So for my family, this is a special-occasion breakfast food (think Christmas, New Year's, etc.). And it's always balanced with veggie juice, protein, and maybe a fruit salad for the kids and a green "brunch salad" for the adults. But as far as breakfast cakes go, this is pretty healthy.

NOTE: If you're gluten-free, use an all-purpose gluten-free flour blend instead of whole wheat pastry flour.

Streusel

2 tablespoons whole wheat pastry flour

½ cup unsweetened shredded dried coconut

¼ cup coconut sugar processed in a coffee grinder or food processor to make it fine

2 tablespoons solid (or semisolid) coconut oil

½ teaspoon ground cinnamon

¼ teaspoon ground cardamom

¼ teaspoon ground ginger

Cake

Coconut oil for greasing the pan

2 cups whole wheat pastry flour

¼ cup coconut sugar, processed in a coffee grinder or food processor to make it fine

2 teaspoons baking powder

½ teaspoon baking soda

¼ teaspoon salt

Optional: pinch of cinnamon, cardamom, and/or ginger

1 cup canned coconut milk (not "lite")

1 teaspoon vanilla extract or almond extract

2 eggs

2 cups fresh or frozen berries or chopped fruit, divided

½ cup sliced almonds or another sliced or chopped nut

1. Preheat oven to 350°F.

2. Lightly grease a 9-inch round cake pan with coconut oil. Set aside.

3. Make streusel: Put 2 tablespoons whole wheat pastry flour, shredded coconut, ¼ cup coconut sugar, solid coconut oil, cinnamon, cardamom, and ginger in a medium bowl and cut together with a fork until well combined and mixture is in large clumps. Set streusel aside.

4. Make cake: Whisk together 2 cups whole wheat pastry flour, ¼ cup coconut sugar, baking powder, baking soda, salt, and optional spices in a large bowl until thoroughly combined. Set aside.

5. In a medium bowl, whisk together coconut milk, vanilla, and eggs, then pour into bowl with dry ingredients and stir until combined. Gently fold in 1 cup of the fruit.

6. Spoon batter into prepared pan. Sprinkle streusel over the top.

7. Scatter the remaining 1 cup of fruit over the streusel and top with the almonds.

8. Bake until a toothpick inserted in center of cake comes out clean, 30 to 40 minutes.

9. Allow cake to cool before removing from pan and transferring to a plate.

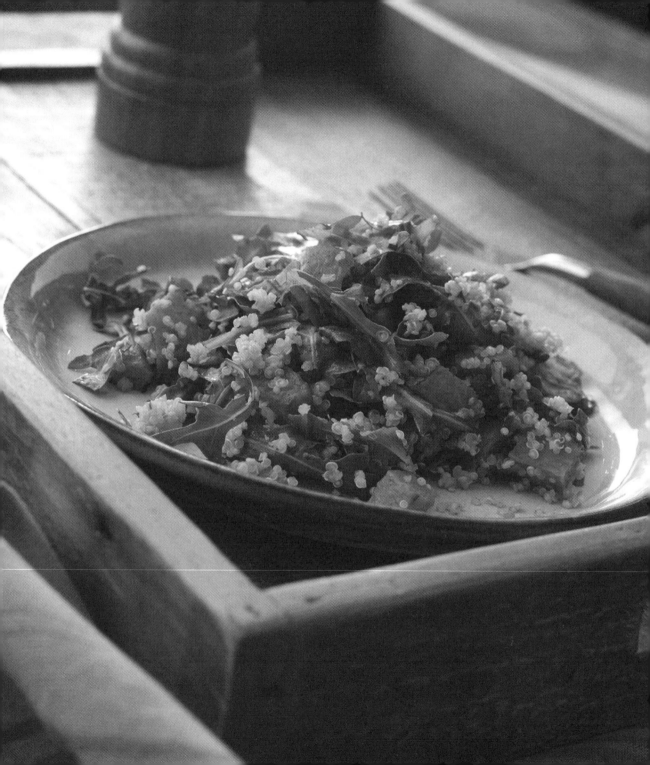

# CHAPTER 5

# COCONUT FOR LUNCH

I believe lunch is essential to a productive, happy afternoon. Your body needs the fuel a midday meal provides to keep you sharp, efficient, and feeling great all day and into the night. And yet, so often, we choose lunch foods not for their health benefits but for their convenience. Here's a fact: What you eat at lunch plays an important role in staying healthy, so let's get used to looking at lunch as a time to replenish nutrient stores and do something to help yourself look and feel great. Fortunately, you can have good nutrition without much fuss. It just takes a bit of planning and a few easy, delicious, nourishing recipes, like the ones in this chapter. This is where I share some of my favorite midday ways to enjoy coconut, with an emphasis on portable, easy-pack foods for those of you who take your lunch to work or school.

## CHILIES, SOUPS, AND STEWS

### SPICED POTAGE

*MAKES 6 SERVINGS*

I love lentils because they contain potassium, calcium, zinc, niacin, and vitamin K—along with exceptionally large amounts of dietary fiber, lean protein, folate, and iron. Together, all of these help keep your energy high and your body's systems working at their best. Add coconut's brain-boosting lauric acid, nutritious veggies, and immune-system-strengthening spices, and wow, you have a great lunchtime dish. Love veggies? Add the leftovers from last night's dinner. You could even reduce the liquid in this recipe to only 3 cups, and make a delicious bean salad to enjoy either all on its own or as a topping for grains and greens.

- 2 tablespoons liquid coconut oil
- 1 medium yellow onion, chopped (1½ cups)
- 1 celery stalk, chopped
- 1 medium carrot, peeled and chopped
- 1 garlic clove, minced
- ½ teaspoon ground ginger
- ½ teaspoon ground turmeric
- ¼ teaspoon ground allspice
- 3 tablespoons tomato paste
- 5 cups vegetable or chicken broth or water, or a mixture

OPPOSITE: **Roasted Sweet Potato, Quinoa, and Arugula Salad, page 89**

1 cup dried French green lentils or regular brown lentils

Pinch of salt

3 teaspoons lime juice

Optional: pepper and additional salt, to taste

**1.** In a large sauté pan over medium heat, warm coconut oil. Add onion, celery, and carrot and sauté until softened, about 7 or 8 minutes.

**2.** Stir in garlic, and cook another minute.

**3.** Stir in ginger, turmeric, and allspice, and sauté 30 seconds.

**4.** Stir in tomato paste and sauté 30 seconds. Add 1 cup of the broth to pan, and scrape up any caramelized vegetables.

**5.** Add lentils and 4 cups of broth. Bring to a boil, then reduce heat to medium-low and cover.

**6.** Simmer 30 minutes.

**7.** Add pinch of salt and simmer uncovered for 10 additional minutes, or until lentils are tender (but not mushy!).

**8.** Stir in lime juice, and season with salt and pepper, if desired.

## RED LENTIL CURRY STEW

*MAKES 4 SERVINGS*

The spices used in curries contain polyphenols that can help protect the body against cancer, diabetes, and heart disease, as well as help reduce blood glucose levels.

2 tablespoons liquid coconut oil

2 garlic cloves, minced

1 tablespoon minced fresh ginger

2 teaspoons mild Madras curry powder (use more if desired)

1 teaspoon ground turmeric

2 cups canned coconut milk

2 cups vegetable or chicken broth or water (or more if you want a thin soup)

1½ cups dried red lentils

2 cups frozen green peas or frozen mixed vegetables (use small-size veggies)

½ cup chopped cashews

¼ cup unsweetened shredded dried coconut

Salt and pepper, to taste

1 tablespoon cilantro, chopped

**1.** Heat oil in large skillet over medium heat, and sauté garlic and ginger about 30 seconds, or until fragrant.

**2.** Stir in curry powder and turmeric and sauté for another 30 seconds.

**3.** Add coconut milk, broth (or water), and red lentils. Reduce heat to medium-low, and cook 15 minutes more, or until lentils are softened.

**4.** Stir in frozen peas, cashews, and coconut, and cook 3 more minutes.

**5.** Remove from heat. Stir in salt, pepper, and cilantro, and serve.

## COCOA CHILI

*MAKES 8 SERVINGS*

I just love chili. Any kind. Not being a native Texan, I don't need to worry about the bean vs. no-bean, meat vs. vegetarian, red vs. white vs. green arguments that seem to arise when people talk about chili. I can just enjoy whatever is put in front of me. I especially like this recipe, which has a slightly smoky taste, thanks to the cocoa and allspice. It features a trio of pinto, kidney, and black beans, all rich in protein and fiber. But feel free to use the same measure of just one of these beans, or try another bean altogether. This chili is nothing if not flexible.

1   tablespoon liquid coconut oil

2   cups diced onion

1   cup celery, diced

½   cup diced jicama or chayote

½   cup red, orange, or yellow bell peppers, diced

6   medium garlic cloves, minced

½   teaspoon salt

    Freshly ground black pepper, to taste

2   tablespoons mild chili powder blend

½   teaspoon cinnamon

⅛   teaspoon allspice

3   tablespoons Dutch-processed cocoa powder

2   28-ounce cans diced tomatoes with liquid

1   14-ounce can black beans, rinsed and drained

1   14-ounce can kidney beans, rinsed and drained

1   14-ounce can pinto beans, rinsed and drained

1   14-ounce can coconut milk

½   cup unsweetened shredded dried coconut

1   cup frozen corn kernels

**1.** In a large soup pot over medium heat, add coconut oil, onion, celery, jicama or chayote, bell pepper, garlic, salt, pepper, chili powder, cinnamon, and allspice and stir to combine. Cover and cook until onions start to soften, about 7 to 9 minutes, stirring occasionally.

**2.** Add cocoa and stir for 1 to 2 minutes.

**3.** Add tomatoes, beans, coconut milk, and shredded coconut, and stir to combine. Increase heat to bring to a boil. Once boiling, reduce heat to low and cover, simmering for 20 to 25 minutes, stirring occasionally.

**4.** Stir in corn kernels, and cook another 5 minutes to heat through.

# COCONUT CHICKEN CHILI

*MAKES 4 SERVINGS*

Okay, so this chili is completely untraditional. It's white. It's made with chicken. And it contains coconut, ginger, nut butter, and basil. It is delicious, filling, and loaded with protein, fiber, and nutrients that support your brain health and immune system. It also gives you a steady drip of energy so that you can make it through the day beautifully. I think you'll like it!

1 *tablespoon liquid coconut oil*

12 *ounces skinless, boneless chicken breast halves, chopped*

1 *large onion, chopped*

1 ½ *teaspoons chili powder*

1 ½ *teaspoons ground ginger*

½ *teaspoon salt*

½ *teaspoon black pepper*

¼ *teaspoon ground cayenne pepper*

1 *tablespoon coconut flour*

1 *14-ounce can coconut milk*

1 *tablespoon peanut butter or other nut butter*

1 *cup water or broth*

1 *15-ounce can cannellini beans, rinsed and drained*

3 *medium carrots, shredded*

1 *stalk celery, sliced*

1 *medium green onion, sliced*

5 *garlic cloves, minced*

2 *tablespoons chopped fresh basil*

**1.** Heat coconut oil in large saucepan over medium heat. Add chicken, onion, chili powder, ginger, salt, black pepper, and cayenne pepper and cook 6 to 8 minutes or until chicken is no longer pink.

**2.** Stir in coconut flour and cook 1 more minute.

**3.** Stir in coconut milk, peanut butter, and water. Bring to a boil, stirring occasionally.

**4.** Stir in beans, carrots, celery, green onion, garlic, and basil. Return to boiling; reduce heat. Simmer, covered, 10 minutes.

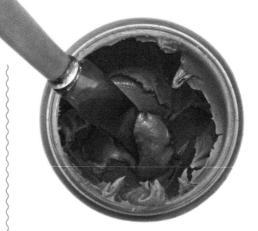

## LUNCH BOWLS

### GINGER MILLET WITH VEGGIES

*MAKES 4 SERVINGS*

Millet is another one of my favorites. This ancient grain nourished centuries of Africans, Asians, and Europeans. Today, most people know it best as a component of birdseed. Fortunately, a growing number of healthy eaters are falling in love with this superfood, both for its nutty flavor and its impressive nutritional profile. Millet boasts protein and fiber, as well as large amounts of magnesium, iron, calcium, phosphorus, and potassium. It contains B-complex vitamins, vitamin E, and amino acids. In this recipe, it's complemented by our superfood friend, coconut, the powerful cruciferous superstar, cabbage, beans, and sunflower seeds.

- 1   *cup millet*
- 2   *to 3 tablespoons minced fresh ginger*
- 1   *teaspoon salt, divided*
- 3   *cups water or broth*
- 3   *tablespoons sesame oil*
- 3   *tablespoons coconut vinegar or apple cider vinegar*
- 1   *15-ounce can black beans, drained and rinsed*
- 2   *tablespoons liquid coconut oil*

- 1   *carrot, finely diced*
- 3   *radishes, finely diced*
- ½   *cup snow peas or sugar snap peas, chopped*
- ½   *cup shredded red cabbage*
- 3   *scallions, thinly sliced*
   *Salt, to taste*
   *Freshly ground black pepper, to taste*
- ¼   *cup sunflower seeds or walnuts or another seed or nut*

**1.** Place millet and ginger in a small saucepan. Add ½ teaspoon salt and the water. Bring to a boil, stir once, then reduce heat and simmer, covered, for 25 minutes.

**2.** As the millet cooks, whisk together sesame oil, vinegar, and remaining ½ teaspoon salt in a large bowl. Set aside.

**3.** Check millet. When it is done, remove from heat and allow to rest for 10 minutes.

**4.** Fluff with a fork and add beans. Set aside.

**5.** Warm coconut oil in a large sauté pan. Flash-sauté carrots, radishes, snow peas, cabbage, and scallions until firm-tender. Season with salt and pepper.

**6.** Spoon sautéed veggies into the bowl with the vinaigrette and stir to coat ingredients.

**7.** Stir in millet-bean mixture and sunflower seeds and continue stirring to coat.

# BLACK RICE SALAD WITH MANGO AND PEANUTS

*MAKES 4 SERVINGS*

If you're not familiar with black rice, let me introduce you: Known also as "forbidden rice," this wonderful, nutty grain features a black bran coating, which gives it outrageously high levels of protein, fiber, and antioxidants, including vitamin E and anthocyanin (which gives the rice its black hue). It is so high in phytonutrients that a study done by Louisiana State University Agricultural Center found that it was more antioxidant-dense than blueberries, one of the darlings of the superfood world. Now that you know a bit about this powerhouse, give this delicious recipe a try! Black rice travels beautifully, making it the perfect lunch food.

- ¾ cup orange juice
- ¼ cup fresh lime juice
- 2 tablespoons liquid coconut oil
- 1 tablespoon coconut aminos or natural soy sauce
  Salt, to taste
- 3½ cups water
- 2 cups black rice
- ½ red, orange, or yellow pepper, seeded and diced
- 2 stalks celery, cut into small dice
- 1 cup fresh cilantro leaves, chopped
- 1 cup finely chopped red onion
- ½ cup unsalted, dry-roasted peanuts
- 6 scallions, thinly sliced
- 1 small firm-ripe mango or avocado, cut into small dice
- 1 jalapeño pepper, seeded and minced

**1.** In a large bowl, whisk together orange juice, lime juice, coconut oil, coconut aminos, and a pinch of salt. Whisk to blend. Set aside.

**2.** In a medium saucepan, heat water to boiling. Season lightly with salt and pour in black rice. Cover, reduce heat to low, and simmer until all liquid is absorbed and rice is tender, about 25 minutes.

**3.** Remove pan from heat and let stand, covered, for 15 minutes.

**4.** As rice stands, add red pepper, celery, cilantro, red onion, peanuts, scallions, mango or avocado, and jalapeño to the large bowl containing dressing. Stir to coat ingredients.

**5.** Add black rice, stirring gently until coated.

**6.** Allow to sit for 30 or more minutes for flavors to blend.

# GRAIN OR BEAN SALAD BLUEPRINT

*MAKES 2 SERVINGS*

Grain salads and bean salads are easy to make, versatile, economical, healthy, and delicious. This blueprint allows you to create your own grain salads and bean salads using what you currently have in your pantry, refrigerator, freezer, and garden. Have fun!

¼ cup (or more) vinaigrette or favorite salad dressing (homemade or store-bought)

1 tablespoon (or more) favorite herb or mix of herbs

1 garlic clove, minced

¼ cup onion, scallions, or shallots

Pinch of salt and pepper

4 cups cooked beans or grain of choice

1 cup chopped cooked or raw vegetables

Optional: 1 cup animal or plant protein of choice

Optional: ¼ cup (or more) nuts or seeds, for crunch

**1.** In a large bowl, whisk together salad dressing, herbs, garlic, onion, salt, and pepper.

**2.** Add in all other ingredients, stirring gently until well coated.

**3.** Adjust salt and pepper to taste.

**4.** Allow to sit for 30 or more minutes so flavors can blend.

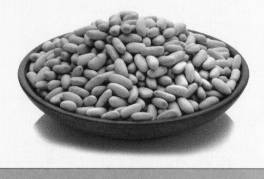

## MEXICALI QUINOA PILAF

*MAKE 2 SERVINGS*

Every ingredient in this one-dish meal contributes a large number of nutrients. Make this pilaf once a week, take it to work, and you will feel energized and alert, while doing wonderful things for your cardiovascular system, nervous system, immune system, and other parts of your body. Feel free to play around with the recipe. Try adding a cup of chopped leftover veggies, use a different type of legume or herb, or add in something else that isn't in the ingredient list.

- 2  *tablespoons coconut oil*
- 2  *garlic cloves, minced*
- ½  *cup diced red, orange, or yellow bell peppers*
- ¼  *teaspoon cayenne powder*
- ¼  *teaspoon chili powder*
- 3  *or more scallions, chopped*
- 15  *ounces black beans, rinsed and drained*
- 1  *14-ounce can coconut milk*
- ½  *cup chopped pepitas (green, hulled pumpkin seeds) or sunflower seeds*
- ¼  *teaspoon salt*
- ¼  *cup chopped cilantro*
- 3  *cups cooked quinoa*

**1.** Preheat oven to 350°F.

**2.** Add the coconut oil to a large skillet over medium heat, and sauté garlic, peppers, cayenne powder, chili powder, and scallions until just tender, about 5 minutes. Remove from heat and set aside.

**3.** In a casserole dish, stir together black beans, coconut milk, pepitas, and salt.

**4.** Stir in the sautéed ingredients, cilantro, and quinoa.

**5.** Bake for 30 minutes, or until top is golden.

## QUINOA BOWL

*MAKES 2 SERVINGS*

Wow, does quinoa contain a lot of protein: 24 g per 1-cup serving! Quinoa also contains generous amounts of fiber, magnesium, manganese, iron, vitamins B2 and B6, lysine, and phytochemicals that help the brain, heart, and immune system. This delicious dish pairs quinoa with coconut, for a portable, nourishing midday nosh.

### WHAT ARE ANTHOCYANINS?

Anthocyanins are antioxidants that have been found to help fight heart disease, diabetes, and Alzheimer's, and are currently being studied for their role in helping fight cancer. Dark blue, red, and purple foods, such as blueberries, acai berries, and black rice are loaded with anthocyanins.

1  tablespoon liquid coconut oil

¼  cup finely diced carrot

¼  cup diced celery

¼  cup diced onion

1  teaspoon grated fresh ginger

½  teaspoon minced garlic

10  peeled and deveined shrimp
    (or 1 cup of cubed chicken or beans)

4  cups cooked quinoa

3  tablespoons unsweetened shredded dried
    coconut

½  tablespoon lime juice
    Optional: cilantro for garnish

**1.** Warm coconut oil in a large sauté pan over medium heat. Add carrot, celery, and onion and sauté until tender.

**2.** Add ginger and garlic and cook for just about a minute.

**3.** Add shrimp and cook until done, being careful not to overcook.

**4.** Remove from heat and stir in quinoa, shredded coconut, and lime juice. Sprinkle with cilantro, if desired.

# CHICKPEA COCONUT SALAD

*MAKES 4 SERVINGS*

This yummy chickpea salad is filled with protein, fiber, and antioxidants—the perfect dish to fuel yourself. You can change things up by adding a cup of chopped, cooked veggies; a tablespoon or more of another chopped herb; a handful of nuts or seeds; or even some dried fruit. I like a cup of this salad on top of a bed of arugula or any other salad green.

1  tablespoon lemon juice

1  tablespoon liquid coconut oil

⅓  cup chopped fresh cilantro

½  teaspoon salt
    Pinch of pepper

1  15-ounce can chickpeas, rinsed and drained

⅓  cup freshly grated coconut
    (or unsweetened shredded dried coconut)

1  teaspoon chopped green chili peppers

**1.** In a large bowl, whisk together lemon juice, coconut oil, cilantro, salt, and pepper.

**2.** Add remaining ingredients and gently stir to coat.

**3.** Allow to sit for at least 30 minutes for flavors to blend.

## LUNCH SALADS

### CHOPPED SUPERFOOD SALAD

*MAKES 6 SERVINGS*

This delicious, chopped salad is a bit different—it's almost a slaw—and contains pectin-rich apple, coconut, cilantro, and other good things that will help boost your energy and good health. You'll like this one! If you leave out the protein, it also makes a great side dish for burgers, hot dogs, or anything barbecued.

- 2 to 3 tablespoons lemon juice
- 1 tablespoon liquid coconut oil
- ½ teaspoon pepper
- 1 teaspoon salt
- 4 cups green cabbage, shredded, and diced into small bits
- 1 crisp apple or Asian pear, cored and diced
- ½ cup walnuts, chopped
- 2 cups chicken, turkey, pork, or favorite bean
- ½ cup fresh cilantro, chopped
- ½ cup unsweetened shredded dried coconut

**1.** In a large bowl, whisk together lemon juice, coconut oil, pepper, and salt.

**2.** Add remaining ingredients and gently stir to coat.

**3.** Allow to sit for at least 30 minutes for flavors to blend.

### KALE AND COCONUT CHICKEN SALAD

*MAKES 2 SERVINGS*

Where would a superfood cookbook—even one on coconut—be without at least one kale recipe? Kale is a member of the Cruciferae family, known for its high antioxidant content, omega-3 fatty acids, protein, and fiber. Here, it teams up with coconut and chicken (or use another animal protein or substitute a cup of legumes), making it a wonderful choice for lunch or a light supper.

- ¼ cup liquid coconut oil
- 1 teaspoon sesame oil (dark sesame oil has the best flavor)
- 2 tablespoons coconut aminos or natural soy sauce
  Dash of salt and pepper
- 5 cups baby kale
- 1 cup unsweetened shredded dried coconut
- 1 cup chicken, cooked and shredded (or substitute 1 cup white beans)

**1.** In a large bowl, whisk together coconut oil, sesame oil, coconut aminos, salt, and pepper.

**2.** Add remaining ingredients and gently stir to coat.

**3.** Allow to sit for at least 30 minutes for flavors to blend.

## CHOPPED AVOCADO COCONUT SALAD

*MAKES 2 SERVINGS*

This recipe is chock-full of nutrient-dense avocado, coconut, fresh herbs, protein, and bold flavor. This is a portable salad, but if you decide to take it to work with you, consider packing the dressing on the side so that the salad stays fresh.

- 1 large Hass avocado, halved, pitted
- 1½ tablespoons fresh lime juice
- 1½ teaspoons Asian chili-garlic sauce, such as sriracha
- 3 tablespoons liquid coconut oil
  Salt and pepper, to taste
- 2 cups diced turkey, chicken, fish, beef, pork, or other animal protein, or a favorite bean
- 1 cup diced peeled jicama
- 1 cup diced red onion
- 1 large red bell pepper, diced
- ¼ cup unsweetened shredded dried coconut
- ¼ cup chopped peanuts or cashews
- ¼ cup chopped fresh cilantro
- 7 cups chopped Romaine lettuce
  Salad dressing of choice

**1.** Scoop avocado flesh into food processor or blender. Add lime juice, chili-garlic sauce, and coconut oil, and process until smooth. Season generously with salt and pepper.

**2.** In a large bowl, toss together remaining ingredients.

**3.** If you are eating right away, pour dressing over salad and toss, toss, toss, until all ingredients are coated in dressing. If you are taking the salad to work, pack dressing separately and dress salad right before eating.

## ROASTED SWEET POTATO, QUINOA, AND ARUGULA SALAD

*MAKES 4 SERVINGS*

Oh my, this is a stunning salad, in an upscale, gourmet, truly yummy kind of way. It's so good for you, too. Sweet potatoes are packed with beta-carotene, arugula contains lutein and zeaxanthin (antioxidants thought to help prevent cancer), and quinoa is the protein-perfect grain-seed that leaves you feeling so energized. Do try this one!

- 1 large sweet potato or beet, peeled and diced (about 2 cups)
- 4 to 5 tablespoons liquid coconut oil, divided
- ½ teaspoon ground cinnamon
  Salt, to taste
- 1 tablespoon freshly squeezed lemon juice
  Pepper, to taste
- 3 cups baby arugula leaves, roughly chopped
- 1½ cups cooked quinoa

1. Preheat oven to 425°F.

2. Prepare a baking sheet with foil or parchment paper.

3. Toss together the sweet potatoes, 2 tablespoons coconut oil, and cinnamon on prepared baking sheet with a pinch of salt.

4. Roast the sweet potatoes until softened and a little bit browned, about 20 minutes.

5. As the sweet potatoes cook, whisk together the remaining coconut oil, lemon juice, salt, and pepper, in a large bowl.

6. When the sweet potatoes are done, allow them to cool slightly on the baking sheet.

7. Add arugula and sweet potato to the dressing and gently toss to coat.

8. Add quinoa and gently combine again, to coat.

## SANDWICHES & WRAPS

## MUSHROOM-BEAN BURGERS

*MAKES 4 SERVINGS*

Mushrooms are popular in the health world as immune-system aids. Here, they are used to give delicious bean burgers a meaty, toothsome texture. And there's lots of protein and fiber here! Leave out the coconut aminos if you don't have any, but its soy sauce–like flavor is nice here.

4   tablespoons liquid coconut oil, divided

1   onion, diced

1   clove garlic, minced

¾   cup diced fresh mushrooms
    Optional: 1 teaspoon coconut aminos

1   15-ounce can pinto beans, or another bean

¼   cup unsweetened shredded dried coconut

1   tablespoon fresh parsley or chives, minced
    Salt and pepper, to taste

2   tablespoons coconut oil

1. Sauté onion and garlic in 2 tablespoons coconut oil for 3 to 5 minutes, until onion is soft. Add mushrooms and coconut aminos, and cook for another 5 minutes, until mushrooms are cooked. Set aside.

2. In a large bowl, mash the beans until slightly chunky.

3. Stir in the coconut, parsley, salt, and pepper until thoroughly combined.

4. Add the mushroom mixture to the beans. Stir until well combined. Allow to sit for 5 minutes or more. (You can cover bowl and come back to mixture later in the day if you'd like.)

5. Shape the mixture into patties. Heat about 2 tablespoons of coconut oil and cook each patty until the veggie burgers are done, about 5 minutes on each side.

## BETTER TUNA SALAD

*MAKES 2 SERVINGS*

A lot of my clients love tuna salad. To create a healthier version, I ask them to replace the mayo with a bit of coconut milk and add lots of veggies. This tuna salad can be eaten on top of salad greens, made into a sandwich or wrap, or packed into a container and used as a dip to enjoy with gluten-free seed crackers, veggie strips, or apple slices. For something different, use salmon or another fish instead of tuna.

2 to 3 tablespoons canned coconut milk, depending upon how moist you like your tuna salad

1 teaspoon apple cider vinegar

1 to 2 teaspoons curry powder

Salt and pepper, to taste

Optional: 1 tablespoon cilantro, parsley, or chives (or a mixture of all three), chopped fine

1 2.5- to 3-ounce can or pouch of tuna (or salmon)

Optional: 1 scallion, chopped fine

Optional: ½ celery stalk, chopped fine

Optional: 1 small carrot, shredded

Optional: ¼ red pepper, chopped fine

Optional: 2 tablespoons sunflower seeds or chopped cashews

**1.** In a large bowl, whisk together coconut milk, vinegar, curry powder, salt, pepper, and if desired, herbs. Adjust spices to taste.

**2.** Stir in tuna until just coated. (Leave chunky.)

**3.** Stir in remaining ingredients until just coated.

## BLACK BEAN BURGERS

*MAKES 4 SERVINGS*

Black beans are loaded with antioxidants, which you can tell from their deep color. They also have plenty of fiber and protein. Garlic, pepper, spices, veggies, and coconut add even more antioxidants, making this burger a delicious way to help your immune system stay strong. Other beans will work beautifully in this recipe, as well.

2 tablespoons liquid coconut oil, or as needed

1 small onion, diced

2 cloves garlic, minced

1 jalapeño pepper, seeded and minced

½ red bell pepper, diced

1 cup fresh or frozen corn kernels

1 15-ounce can black beans, drained

⅓ cup gluten-free, whole wheat, or regular bread crumbs

¼ cup unsweetened shredded dried coconut

3 teaspoons chili powder blend

1 teaspoon ground cumin

½ teaspoon salt

Pinch of black pepper

½ cup gluten-free or all-purpose flour, or as needed

**1.** Heat 1 tablespoon of the coconut oil in a skillet over medium heat. Add onion, garlic, and jalapeño pepper, stirring occasionally until onion is translucent, 8 to 10 minutes.

**2.** Add red pepper and corn and sauté another 3 or 4 minutes, until red pepper is tender. Remove from heat and set aside.

**3.** In a large bowl, mash black beans until chunky.

**4.** Stir in vegetable mixture, bread crumbs, coconut, chili powder, cumin, salt, and black pepper. Allow to sit for 5 minutes or longer. (You can cover bowl and come back to mixture later in the day if you'd like.)

**5.** Divide mixture into 4 patties and coat both sides of each patty with flour.

**6.** Heat 1 tablespoon coconut oil in a skillet over medium heat; cook patties until browned, about 7 to 8 minutes on each side.

## COCONUT CURRY CHICKEN WRAPS

*MAKES 4 SERVINGS*

This yummy wrap goes heavy on the veggies for a nutrient-rich lunch. Feel free to leave out an ingredient or substitute any veggies or nuts you'd like. You can even use a different animal protein if you'd prefer (turkey, pork, and beef work well). Buy green curry paste in most well-stocked supermarkets.

½ cup canned coconut milk

1 tablespoon Thai green curry paste

1 teaspoon lime or lemon juice

Pinch of salt

Pinch of pepper

2 tablespoons chopped fresh cilantro

1¼ cups shredded cooked chicken

¼ cup shredded carrot

¼ cup very thinly sliced red pepper

2 tablespoons thinly sliced green onion

2 tablespoons chopped roasted peanuts or cashews

4 8-inch tortillas or wraps

1 cup shredded lettuce or cabbage

¼ cup unsweetened shredded dried coconut

**1.** In a medium bowl, whisk together coconut milk, curry paste, lime juice, salt, and pepper until smooth.

**2.** Stir in cilantro, chicken, carrot, red pepper, green onion, and peanuts and toss to coat.

**3.** Arrange tortillas in a single layer on a flat surface. Place ¼ of chicken mixture down the center of each tortilla.

**4.** Top with lettuce and a sprinkle of shredded coconut.

**5.** Roll up tortillas burrito-style and tuck in the ends snugly.

**6.** If desired, halve each wrap crosswise. Serve immediately or wrap tightly in plastic wrap and refrigerate until ready to eat.

# MAKE YOUR OWN WRAP

Did you know you can make your own wraps using healthy coconut? It's actually easy. Give these two a go. I think you'll like them.

## SIMPLE COCONUT WRAP

*MAKES 1 OR 2 SERVINGS*

3   egg whites

½   tablespoon coconut flour

    Pinch of salt

    *Optional: herbs, spices, or extracts to flavor the wraps*

    *Small amount of liquid coconut oil*

**1.** Place all ingredients except the coconut oil in a food processor or high-power blender (such as a Vitamix or Blendtec). Process until ingredients form a smooth batter.

**2.** Coat a large skillet with a very thin layer of coconut oil. Heat over medium heat.

**3.** When skillet is completely heated, pour mixture into skillet and swirl to spread evenly over entire surface of pan. Cover pan.

**4.** Let wrap cook for 1 or 2 minutes; it may puff up, which is fine.

**5.** Uncover pan and, using a large pancake turner, flip the wrap.

**6.** Cook another 30 seconds and slide onto plate or other flat surface.

## PALEO TORTILLAS

*MAKES 3 SERVINGS*

2   eggs

1   teaspoon liquid coconut oil

1   tablespoon water or unflavored coconut water

¼   cup arrowroot powder

1   teaspoon coconut flour

    Dash of salt

    *Optional: herbs, spices, or extracts to flavor the wraps*

**1.** In a medium bowl, whisk the eggs.

**2.** Whisk in the coconut oil and water.

**3.** Add arrowroot powder, coconut flour, salt, and optional flavorings. Stir well to combine.

**4.** In a small skillet over medium heat, pour in about ⅓ of the batter and immediately roll it around to evenly coat the bottom. Cook about 1 minute, or until tortilla begins to pull away from the pan's edges.

**5.** Flip and cook another minute, or until done.

**6.** Use immediately or cool and store in a plastic bag or airtight container.

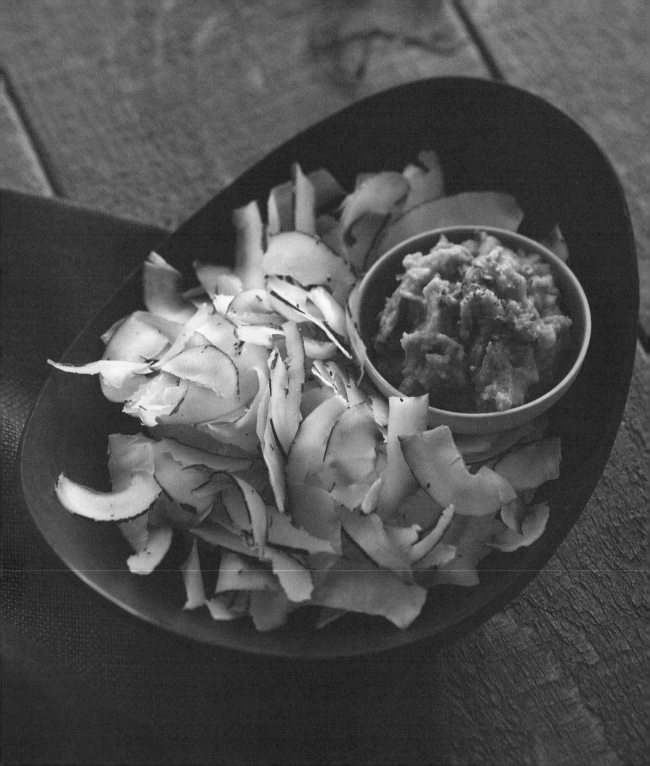

# CHAPTER 6

# SMALL BITES: COCONUT APPETIZERS AND SNACKS

Sometimes you just want a little something—a snack or something fancy before a dinner party so you can show off your ingenious culinary skills. Then there are the times when your kids come home from school or soccer practice absolutely famished, and you want something yummy and healthy to offer them.

Instead of something out of a bag, think coconut. Yes, coconut! Coconut is so versatile that it lends itself to a wide variety of appetizers, sandwiches, dips, and more. Get creative. Try the recipes in this section and then start improvising. I'm sure you'll come up with all kinds of delicious coconut munchies.

## CHIPS, CRISPS, AND CRACKERS

### COCONUT SEED CRACKERS

*MAKES 20 TO 25 CRACKERS*

If you're handy with a rolling pin, this nutritious recipe is great fun to make with kids! Try serving these crackers with one of the dips or spreads from this section.

*½ cup almond flour*
*½ cup macadamia nuts*
*1 tablespoon coconut flour*
*¼ cup pumpkin seeds*
*2 tablespoons sunflower seeds*
*2 tablespoons sesame seeds*
*2 tablespoons hemp seeds*
*1 tablespoon chia seeds*
*1 tablespoon unsweetened shredded dried coconut*
*½ teaspoon salt*
*1 tablespoon coconut oil*
*¼ cup coconut water or regular water*

**1.** Pulse almond flour, macadamias, and coconut flour in a food processor until thoroughly ground.

**2.** Pulse in seeds, dried coconut, and salt until almost fully ground (leave a little texture for crunch).

**3.** Pulse in oil, then coconut water, until dough forms a ball.

**4.** Tightly wrap dough in plastic wrap or put in an airtight container and place in the refrigerator for 30 minutes or longer.

**5.** Preheat oven to 300°F.

**6.** Remove dough from refrigerator and roll out between 2 pieces of wax paper or parchment paper. Roll dough to ¼-inch thickness, or thinner if you prefer.

**7.** Using a sharp knife or a pizza cutter, cut dough into 2-inch squares.

**8.** Gently place crackers on a baking sheet (or sheets) lined with parchment paper or foil.

**9.** Bake for 20 to 25 minutes. Do not overcook; crackers should be golden around the edges. (They will firm up as they cool.)

**10.** Allow crackers to cool thoroughly before removing them from the pan.

## GOLDEN RICE CRISPS

*MAKES 4 APPETIZER SERVINGS*

Since rice flour varies in texture, depending upon the manufacturer, go ahead and use what is convenient for you. Silky, finely milled rice flour will produce thin crisps. Slightly coarser, grittier flour makes thicker crisps. They are all delicious! Just one word of warning: Avoid sweet or glutinous rice flour—it is a different animal!

*½ cup brown or white rice flour (if using finely milled rice flour, use 1 ½ to 2 tablespoons less water)*

*¼ cup cornstarch*

*½ teaspoon ground dried turmeric*

*1 cup coconut water or regular water*

*¼ cup canned coconut milk*

*2 tablespoons thinly sliced green onion, including tops*

*1 tablespoon coconut oil*

**1.** Preheat oven to 350°F.

**2.** In a bowl, mix rice flour, cornstarch, and turmeric. Add coconut water and coconut milk, and whisk to blend. Stir in green onion.

**3.** Set a 12-inch nonstick frying pan (about 10 inches across bottom) over high heat. When pan is hot, add 1 teaspoon oil and tilt to coat bottom.

**4.** Pour ½ cup batter into pan all at once and tilt pan to cover entire bottom evenly.

**5.** Cook until crisp is browned and crunchy on the bottom, 3 to 5 minutes.

**6.** Using a wide spatula, so the crisp doesn't break, transfer to a large baking sheet. Repeat in order to make 2 more crisps, being careful to avoid stacking crisps on top of each other.

**7.** Transfer baking sheet (or sheets) to oven and bake until crisps are completely crisp, about 8 to 12 minutes. Transfer to racks to cool.

**8.** Break off pieces of the crisps and dip them into one of the relishes, salsas, or chutneys in this chapter.

**NOTE:** Crisps can be made up to 1 day ahead and stored in an airtight container in a cool place. To re-crisp, heat, uncovered, in a 350°F oven until crisp again, about 5 minutes.

## COCONUT CHIPS USING A MATURE COCONUT

*MAKES 4 SERVINGS*

You can buy a small pouch of coconut chips at the supermarket for $4.99, or you can make your own.

**NOTE:** Dogs love these chips, so guard them well if you happen to be a pet owner who doesn't want to share.

1   *mature coconut*
    *Coarse salt*

**1.** Preheat oven to 350°F.

**2.** Test each of the three eyes at stem end of coconut to see which two are the softest. Then use a clean ice pick (or a screwdriver or large nail) and a clean hammer to pierce two of the eyes. Or pierce soft eyes with a corkscrew.

**3.** Strain the coconut water through a fine sieve into a bowl; reserve it for other uses (there are plenty of ideas in this book!).

**4.** Place coconut on a rimmed baking sheet; bake for 30 minutes, or until coconut shell begins to crack. Set aside until cool enough to handle.

**5.** Wrap coconut in a clean kitchen towel. Holding coconut with one hand, hit it with a hammer in the same place several times to crack the outer shell and split the coconut into several large pieces.

**6.** Separate coconut flesh from shell, and use a vegetable peeler to remove the dark outer skin, if desired. Rinse coconut in a colander, then spread in a single layer on a kitchen towel to dry.

**7.** Divide coconut strips between 2 rimmed baking sheets in a single layer. Season with salt.

**8.** Bake until toasted, about 10 minutes.

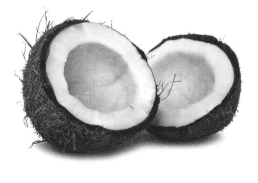

## DIPS & SPREADS

### AVOCADO-COCONUT DIP

*MAKES ABOUT 1½ CUPS*

I think of this dip as "coconut-kissed" guacamole. It is filled with healthy fats from both the avocado and the coconut cream, making it a nourishing (and delicious) superfood dip.

- 3 tablespoons coconut cream or coconut milk, at room temperature
- 1 tablespoon fresh lemon or lime juice
- 1 ripe avocado
  Salt, to taste
  Black pepper, to taste

**1.** In a small bowl, thoroughly mix coconut cream and lemon juice.

**2.** In a separate bowl, mash avocado until smooth.

**3.** Mix avocado into coconut-lemon mixture and season to taste with salt and pepper.

### COCONUT CHUTNEY

*MAKES ABOUT 1 CUP*

I love chutney as a spread on sandwiches, a relish for pork, a dip with veggie slices or crackers, and a burger topping, as well as mixed into grains. This lovely chutney recipe features our beloved coconut.

- 1 cup unsweetened shredded dried or fresh-grated coconut
- 3 tablespoons dry-roasted cashews or peanuts (or a combination)
- 1 teaspoon grated fresh ginger (use a box grater or microplane grater)
- 2 fresh small mild serrano or jalapeño chilies, roughly chopped
- ¼ cup chopped cilantro leaves
- 1 teaspoon salt
- ¼ teaspoon coconut sugar
  Optional: ½ teaspoon coconut vinegar or apple cider vinegar (if you like a tangy chutney)
- ⅓ cup coconut water or water
- 1 tablespoon liquid coconut oil
- 1 teaspoon black mustard seeds

**1.** Put coconut, cashews, ginger, chilies, cilantro, salt, coconut sugar, and if desired, vinegar in a blender or food processor. Process, adding coconut water a little at a time, until paste has a smooth consistency. Transfer to a small mixing bowl and set aside.

**2.** Heat coconut oil in a small skillet over medium heat. Add mustard seeds and cook just until they begin to pop. Remove pan from heat and stir the seeds and oil into the chutney.

**3.** Serve immediately or store for up to a week in the refrigerator in a covered container.

# SWEET POTATO & HEMP SEED DIP

*MAKES ABOUT 4 CUPS*

This high-yield recipe is both delicious and versatile—you can use it as a lighter alternative to hummus, as a lovely sandwich spread, or as a fun topping for burritos and tacos. Plus, it is a great way to get concentrated doses of phytonutrients; vitamins A, C, and E; healthy fats; fiber; and protein.

- *4 cups sweet potato, peeled and cubed*
- *4 cups cauliflower florets*
- *1 tablespoon liquid coconut oil*
- *1 medium white onion, chopped*
- *5 cloves garlic*
- *½ to 1 teaspoon chipotle chili powder*
- *2 teaspoons cumin powder*
- *4 tablespoons lime juice (from about two limes)*
- *¼ cup coconut yogurt*
- *¼ cup unsweetened shredded dried coconut*
- *Salt, to taste*
- *Ground black pepper, to taste*
- *⅓ cup hempseed*
- *¼ to ⅓ cup cilantro, chopped*

**1.** Bring a large pot of salted water to a boil. Place the cubed sweet potatoes and cauliflower florets in the pot. Cover and cook the vegetables until they have completely softened, about 15 to 20 minutes.

**2.** Drain the cooked vegetables in a colander and allow to cool slightly.

**3.** While the vegetables are cooling, heat the coconut oil in a skillet on medium-high heat. Sauté the chopped onion for 4 to 5 minutes, until golden brown. Then, add garlic and continue to sauté for 30 to 40 seconds. Remove from heat and transfer to a food processor.

**4.** Add the cooked vegetables, chipotle powder, cumin powder, lime juice, coconut yogurt, shredded coconut, salt, and pepper to the food processor. Process until almost smooth (scraping the sides of the processor may be necessary).

**5.** Add the hempseed and pulse until completely mixed. Taste and adjust seasonings, if required.

**6.** Garnish the dip with chopped cilantro.

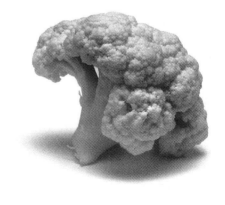

## FRESH COCONUT RELISH

*MAKES 1⅓ CUPS*

This is a souped-up, cucumber-free, purely coconut version of that Indian favorite: raita. It is super-healthful, and so delicious and different that you'll have people clamoring for the recipe. This relish also gives you something to make with fresh coconut meat. (Use meat from a brown, or mature, coconut for this recipe. The flesh of a young green coconut is too gelatinous to work well here.)

- 1 *cup packed fresh grated coconut from a mature coconut*
- ½ *cup plain (unsweetened) coconut yogurt*
  *Optional: 2 tablespoons finely chopped cilantro leaves*
- 2 *small mild green chilies, such as a mild jalapeño*
- ½ *teaspoon salt*
- 2 *tablespoons hot water*
- 4 *tablespoons liquid coconut oil*
- 1 *teaspoon black mustard seeds*

**1.** Put coconut, yogurt, cilantro (if desired), chilies, salt, and hot water into a food processor or blender and process until finely pureed. Scrape into a medium-size mixing bowl.

**2.** Heat the coconut oil over medium-high heat in a small frying pan. When it is very hot, carefully add the black mustard seeds. (The seeds may sizzle, so keep a lid handy.)

**3.** When the seeds stop spluttering and turn gray, immediately pour the oil and seeds over the coconut puree. Mix thoroughly, adjust salt to taste, and serve.

**NOTE:** This relish may be prepared in advance and refrigerated for up to 2 days. Remove from refrigerator at least 15 minutes before serving.

## GREEN COCONUT PULP CHUTNEY

*MAKES ALMOST 1 CUP*

Have you just purchased a young coconut for the water? Are you now wondering what to do with the pulp? Here's a scrumptious idea: Make chutney! This spicy relish can be used as a condiment for Indian food, on burgers and sandwiches, as a dip, as a spread, and more.

- ½ *teaspoon cumin seeds*
- ½ *teaspoon black mustard seeds*
- 1 *cup loosely packed cilantro*
- ¼ *cup onion, chopped*
- ½ *cup fresh coconut pulp from a young (green) coconut*
- 1 *½-inch piece of ginger, roughly chopped*
- 2 *serrano or mild jalapeño chilies*
- 5 *tablespoons lemon juice*
  *Salt, to taste*

1. In a heavy pan over medium heat, toast the cumin and mustard seeds by stirring them or shaking the pan to keep them from burning. When they have slightly darkened in color and smell fragrant, remove from heat and allow to cool.

2. Put the cool cumin and mustard seeds in a clean coffee grinder, spice grinder, or blender and pulse until seeds are pulverized.

3. Add pulverized spices and all other ingredients to a food processor or blender and process until smooth. If needed, add water to thin the chutney.

4. Serve immediately or store for up to a week in the refrigerator in a covered container

## ISLAND SALSA

*MAKES 2 ½ CUPS*

This particular recipe is one of the most unusual and delicious in my collection, thanks to the coconut and peanuts. It is also rich in enzymes, high in vitamins C and A, and contains plenty of protein and fiber. Enjoy with tortilla chips or any of the crackers in this chapter. It also works beautifully as a topping for fish, poultry, or pork.

1 ½ cups chopped fresh or canned pineapple (if canned, drain and save juice)

1 cup chopped mango

¼ cup peanuts or cashews (roasted or raw, salted or unsalted), chopped

¼ cup unsweetened shredded dried coconut

1 cup pineapple juice (or orange juice or a mixture)

¼ cup canned coconut milk (not "lite")

½ small red bell pepper, diced

¼ cup red onion, diced

2 tablespoons fresh cilantro, chopped

½ teaspoon grated lime zest

2 tablespoons fresh lime juice

1 teaspoon coconut sugar
   Salt, to taste

¼ teaspoon ground ginger

¼ teaspoon ground red or black pepper

1. Stir together pineapple, mango, peanuts, and coconut.

2. In a separate bowl, stir together the rest of the ingredients. Add to pineapple mixture, and toss to coat.

3. Chill 30 minutes.

## NIBBLES

### COCONUT KETTLE CORN

*MAKES APPROXIMATELY 16 CUPS*

I like homemade, cooked-in-coconut-oil popcorn. It provides fiber, it's low in calories, and it's economical. (All of which are important to me.) When my family wants a little sweetness, I make kettle corn. Try it. It's easy!

- ½ *cup liquid coconut oil*
- ½ *cup popcorn kernels*
- ¼ *cup coconut sugar*
- 1 *teaspoon salt*

**1.** In a medium stockpot or large saucepan, heat coconut oil over medium heat. Add 2 or 3 kernels. When kernels pop, add remaining popcorn kernels and sugar, cover pot, and shake continuously.

**2.** Once popping slows down, remove from heat. Let kernels finish popping, then pour into a bowl and toss with salt before serving. Serve immediately.

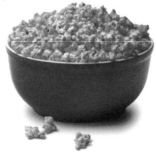

## INDIAN SPICED COCO-NUTS

*MAKES 2 CUPS*

You can easily pack snack-size portions into small bags and tuck them into a purse or lunch box, or you can serve them at your next party—they're that good!

- 1 *cup unsalted peanuts or cashews (preferably unroasted)*
- 1 *cup pecans or walnuts, roughly chopped*
- ¼ *cup unsweetened shredded dried coconut*
- 2 *tablespoons liquid coconut oil*
- 2 *teaspoons ground cumin*
- 2 *teaspoons ground coriander*
- 2 *teaspoons garam masala curry powder*
- *Salt, to taste*

**1.** Preheat oven to 250°F.

**2.** Line a baking sheet with parchment paper.

**3.** In a medium bowl, mix the nuts, shredded coconut, coconut oil, cumin, coriander, garam masala, and salt and pour onto the prepared baking sheet.

**4.** Bake 20 minutes. Open oven and stir nuts.

**5.** Bake another 20 minutes, or until nuts are golden. Do not let nuts burn.

**6.** Remove nuts from oven and allow to cool on the baking sheet.

**7.** Store in an airtight container at room temperature for up to 2 weeks.

## ROASTED COCONUT CHICKPEAS

*MAKES 4 SERVINGS*

Roasted chickpeas are an easy-to-make, protein-rich, fiber-filled, outrageously healthy snack. Most are flavored with salt and spices. This recipe is sweet, though you could omit the sugar, increase the salt by a couple of pinches, and add your favorite savory spices.

1   *15-ounce can chickpeas, rinsed and drained*

1   *tablespoon liquid coconut oil*

1   *tablespoon coconut sugar*

½   *teaspoon salt*

1   *teaspoon ground cinnamon or ½ teaspoon allspice*

  *Optional: pinch of black pepper*

**1.** Preheat oven to 450°F.

**2.** Thoroughly dry chickpeas with paper towels. If necessary, aim a blow-dryer, set to "low cool," on the chickpeas to help get rid of any excess moisture. The beans need to be dry.

**3.** Place chickpeas in a single layer on 1 or 2 baking trays. Roast for 15 minutes.

**4.** Remove from the oven and, while still warm, toss in a large bowl with coconut oil, coconut sugar, salt, spice, and if desired, pepper, making sure all beans are fully coated.

**5.** Return chickpeas to the baking trays and oven. Roast for an additional 15 to 20 minutes until crunchy and golden.

## SMALL BITES

## SATAY SAUCE

*MAKES 1 CUP*

This easy sauce is just as good with meat as it is with vegetables. Use it with the satay in this chapter. Any leftover sauce tastes great over noodles, stirred into grains, or used as a vegetable topper.

2   *teaspoons red curry paste (Thai Kitchen is one brand commonly found in supermarkets)*

1½   *cups canned coconut milk*

½   *cup natural peanut butter*

  *Optional: 1 teaspoon tamarind paste*

  *Salt, to taste*

¼   *cup finely chopped fresh cilantro leaves*

**1.** Heat red curry paste and coconut milk in a wok or heavy saucepan over medium-low heat, stirring for 1 minute.

**2.** Add peanut butter, tamarind paste (if desired), and salt. Lower heat; simmer 10 minutes, stirring constantly.

**3.** Remove from heat and add cilantro.

**4.** Serve with beef, chicken, and other satays or roast meats, or enjoy as a sauce for noodles or veggies.

# CHICKPEA CAKES

*MAKES 4 SERVINGS*

These falafel-like treats are rich in protein and filled with healthy fiber, making them a terrific meatless snack. Serve them with your favorite sauce, salsa, chutney, or relish—any of the ones in this chapter would be fantastic.

- 1   cup dried chickpeas
- 3   tablespoons coconut oil
- ½   cup chopped onion
- ½   cup chopped celery
- 2   tablespoons chopped fresh Italian parsley
- 1   teaspoon sea salt
- 1   teaspoon ground cumin
- ⅓   cup gluten-free all-purpose baking flour (or whole wheat pastry or spelt flour)
- 1   cup finely shredded unsweetened dried coconut
- 2   tablespoons coconut oil

**1.** Put the dried chickpeas in a bowl and add water to cover by about 3 inches. Soak overnight. Drain and rinse.

**2.** In a sauté pan, heat the 3 tablespoons of coconut oil over medium heat. Add the onion and the celery and sauté until softened, about 5 minutes.

**3.** Put the chickpeas, parsley, salt, and cumin into a food processor, and pulse until ground.

**4.** Add the gluten-free flour and pulse a few more times to mix. Don't overprocess: You want a very chunky mixture. Add a tablespoon or more of water if the mixture seems too dry and is not sticking together.

**5.** Transfer mixture to a large bowl and fold in sautéed onion and celery. With your hands, fold the mixture into patties.

**6.** Dredge each patty in the unsweetened shredded dried coconut to coat the entire patty.

**7.** Line a baking sheet with a silicone baking mat or foil. Place patties on the baking sheet and refrigerate for 30 minutes to firm them up.

**8.** Heat the 2 tablespoons of the coconut oil in a sauté pan. Add a few of the chickpea patties and fry until golden brown, about 4 minutes per side. (Alternately, you can bake the patties in a 350°F oven for 10 minutes per side.) Transfer cooked chickpea cakes to a platter lined with paper towels.

**9.** Repeat with remaining chickpea cakes.

# COCONUT LETTUCE TACOS

*MAKES 4 SERVINGS*

This unusual "taco" appetizer is easy, different, and addictive. As an assistant, I learned a version of this recipe years ago from a cooking teacher. You'll have fun with it, too!

**Coconut Filling:**

1   tablespoon coconut oil, melted
    Salt, to taste
1   teaspoon coconut nectar
½   teaspoon smoked paprika
¼   teaspoon ground chipotle
¾   cup unsweetened large coconut shreds

**Coconut Dressing:**

⅓   cup fresh lemon or lime juice
½   cup canned coconut milk
⅔   cup hempseed
4   cloves garlic
1   teaspoon black peppercorns
1   teaspoon salt
⅓   cup coconut oil

**Taco Wraps:**

8   butter lettuce leaves
    Optional: 1 cup leftover shredded chicken, flaked cooked fish, or chopped cooked shrimp
    Optional: 1 or more avocados, diced
    Optional: 1 or more tomatoes, diced

**1.** To make the coconut filling, combine the melted coconut oil, salt, coconut nectar, paprika, and chipotle in a medium bowl and mix well. Add coconut flakes and toss well to evenly coat.

**2.** For the coconut dressing: Combine lemon juice, coconut milk, hempseed, garlic, peppercorns, and salt in a high-speed blender and blend until smooth. While the blender is running, add the ⅓ cup coconut oil and blend. Add water to thin the dressing, if necessary.

**3.** To assemble tacos, lay lettuce leaves on a flat surface or plate. Top each lettuce leaf with a tablespoon of coconut dressing. If desired, add a thin layer of chicken and/or a layer of avocado and tomato.

**4.** Divide the spicy coconut filling among the lettuce leaves, place on individual plates or a platter, and serve.

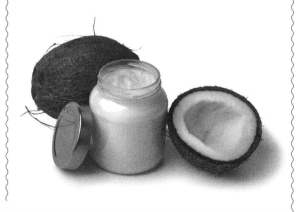

# CURRIED QUINOA CARROT CAKES

*MAKES 4 SERVINGS*

These gluten-free quinoa and carrot "cakes" are a modern take on traditional flavors from India. Try them by themselves, tucked into wraps or pita bread, placed atop salad, or as vegetarian burgers.

- 1  cup uncooked quinoa (rinsed and well drained)
- 2  cups water or mixture of canned coconut milk and water
- ½  teaspoon salt, plus more for seasoning to taste
- ⅓  cup coconut flour
- 1¼ tablespoons mild curry powder
- 1  teaspoon chili powder
- 2  cloves garlic, minced
- 1½ cups carrots, grated (I use the carrot pulp from my juicer after making carrot juice)
- 2  eggs, beaten
- ½  cup cilantro, finely chopped
   Ground black pepper, to taste
- 2  to 4 tablespoons coconut oil (for shallow frying)

**1.** Add the rinsed quinoa, water (or water–coconut milk mixture), and ½ teaspoon salt to a medium-size pot. Cover and bring to a boil. Turn the heat down to a simmer, cover, and cook for 15 minutes.

**2.** Fluff cooked quinoa with a fork, then transfer to a shallow plate or platter for faster cooling. Let cool for 5 minutes.

**3.** While the quinoa is cooling, whisk together coconut flour, curry powder, and chili powder in a large bowl.

**4.** Stir into the coconut flour mixture the cooled quinoa, along with minced garlic, grated carrots, eggs, cilantro, and salt and pepper to taste. Mix well by hand until everything is evenly distributed and there are no lumps of coconut flour remaining.

**5.** With your hands, shape the mixture into 2-inch-wide patties and lay them on a lightly greased plate or baking sheet.

**6.** Heat the coconut oil in a large skillet over medium-high heat. Once the oil is hot, gently add 3 or 4 patties, being careful not to crowd the pan.

**7.** Fry patties on medium heat for 2 to 4 minutes until golden brown. Then turn the cakes and cook on the other side for 2 to 4 minutes. Transfer to a plate lined with a paper towel.

**8.** Repeat with remaining patties.

# SATAY

*MAKES 6 SERVINGS*

When my two older children were born, my husband and I ate a lot of Mexican, Indian, and West Indian (especially Jamaican, Trinidadian, and Bajan) foods. There came a time when we realized we needed to expand the kids' palates a bit, so we ventured into Southeast Asian cooking. Satay was the first Thai dish we served the boys. They loved it! Try serving it with Island Salsa (see page 101) or Satay Sauce (see page 103). I think you'll love it, too.

- 1  *pound chicken breast, London broil, top round beef, or lamb*
- ⅔  *cup canned coconut milk*
- 1  *piece (1 inch) fresh ginger, peeled and grated*
- 2  *tablespoons green curry paste (Thai Kitchen is a brand commonly found in supermarkets)*
- 1  *tablespoon coconut aminos or natural soy sauce*
- 2  *tablespoons coconut oil*
     *Lime wedges, for serving*

**1.** Slice the meat into ⅛-inch-thick strips.

**2.** In a large bowl combine the coconut milk, ginger, green curry paste, and coconut aminos.

**3.** Add the chicken (or beef or lamb) and toss to coat. Cover and chill for 3 hours.

**4.** Meanwhile, in a bowl of water, soak 24 wooden skewers for 30 minutes.

**5.** Thread 1 strip of the meat onto each skewer, weaving in and out at 1-inch intervals.

**6.** Preheat a barbecue grill to high heat or place a grill pan over medium-high heat. Rub the meat lightly with coconut oil and grill, turning once until no longer pink, about 45 seconds per side. Serve with lime wedges.

## YUMMY THINGS TO DO WITH GINGER

- Spice things up by grating a bit of ginger into your next pot of millet, rice, quinoa, or other grain. This is especially delicious served with curries and stir-fry dishes.

- Make ginger lemonade by simply combining freshly grated ginger, lemon juice, cane juice or honey, and water.

- Perk up bottled salad dressing or a simple homemade vinaigrette with grated ginger.

- Add dry powdered or grated fresh ginger to pureed sweet potatoes. A squirt of lemon juice is a yummy addition.

- Add zing to your next fruit salad with some grated ginger.

- Dress up sautéed veggies by tossing in ½ teaspoon of minced fresh ginger.

## BAKED COCONUT SHRIMP

*MAKES 6 SERVINGS*

My younger son, Anders, loves shrimp. He also adores coconut. Being an adventurous eater, he is always looking for new ways to enjoy both foods. This recipe is one of his favorites. We love it with a fruity salsa, but it's also great with chutney, peanut sauce, or a habanero-based hot sauce.

2  *large eggs*

⅓  *cup all-purpose gluten-free or regular flour*

1½  *teaspoons paprika*

½  *teaspoon garlic powder*

1¼  *cups unsweetened dried shredded coconut*

¾  *teaspoon salt*

1  *pound raw shrimp (21 to 25 per pound)*

**1.** Lightly grease a baking sheet. Set aside.

**2.** In a small bowl, beat eggs.

**3.** In another bowl, whisk together flour, paprika, and garlic powder.

**4.** In a third bowl, combine coconut and salt.

**5.** Peel shrimp, leaving the tails on. Butterfly the shrimp by cutting halfway through the back, and stopping at the tail, so the shrimp will stand tail up.

**6.** Grabbing a shrimp by the tail, dredge it in the flour mixture. Dip it in the egg. Then coat the shrimp with coconut, leaving the tail uncoated. Stand the shrimp tail up on the prepared baking sheet. Discard any unused dipping mixtures.

### BUYING SHRIMP

• Shrimp is usually sold by the pound. A "21 to 25 count" means there will be 21 to 25 shrimp in a pound.

• In the shrimp world, sizes, such as "large" and "extra large," are not standardized, so to get the amount you want, order by the count per pound.

• Both wild-caught and farm-raised shrimp can potentially damage the surrounding ecosystems when not managed properly. Buy shrimp that have been raised or caught with sound environmental practices. Look for fresh or frozen shrimp certified by an independent agency, such as the Marine Stewardship Council.

• If you can't find certified shrimp, choose wild-caught shrimp from North America. It is more likely to have been sustainably caught than shrimp harvested in Asia.

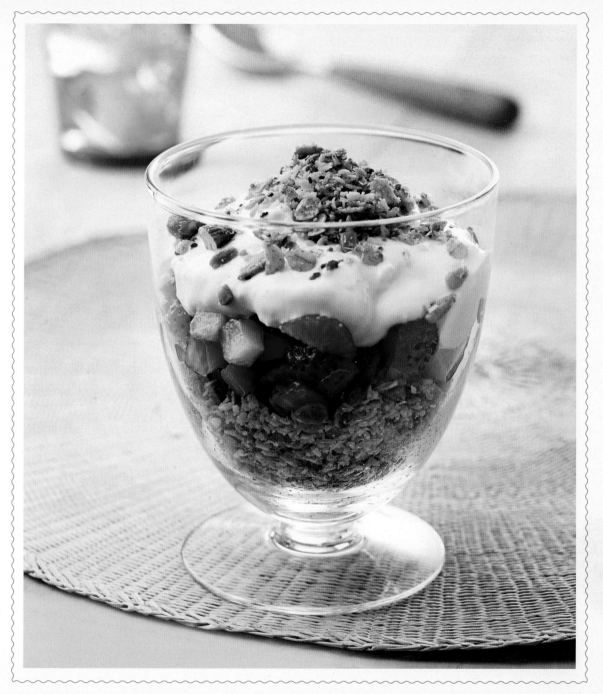

Coconut Granola, page 64

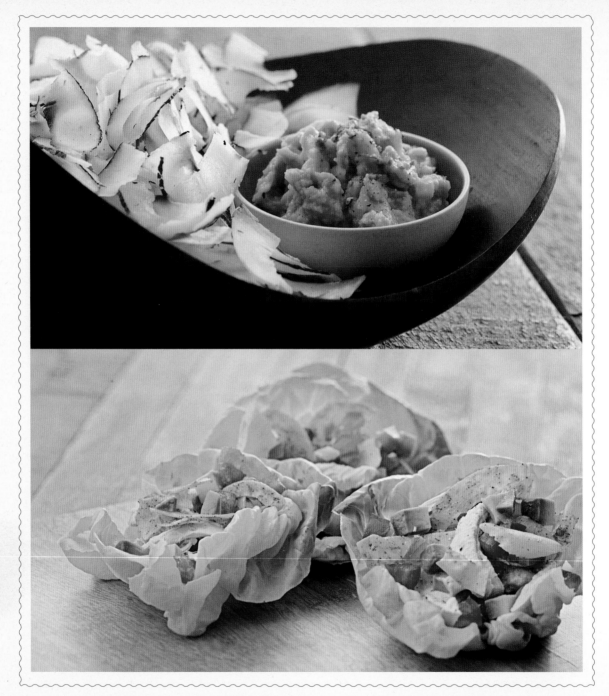

TOP: Coconut Chips Using a Mature Coconut, page 97, and Avocado-Coconut Dip, page 98
BOTTOM: Coconut Lettuce Tacos, page 105

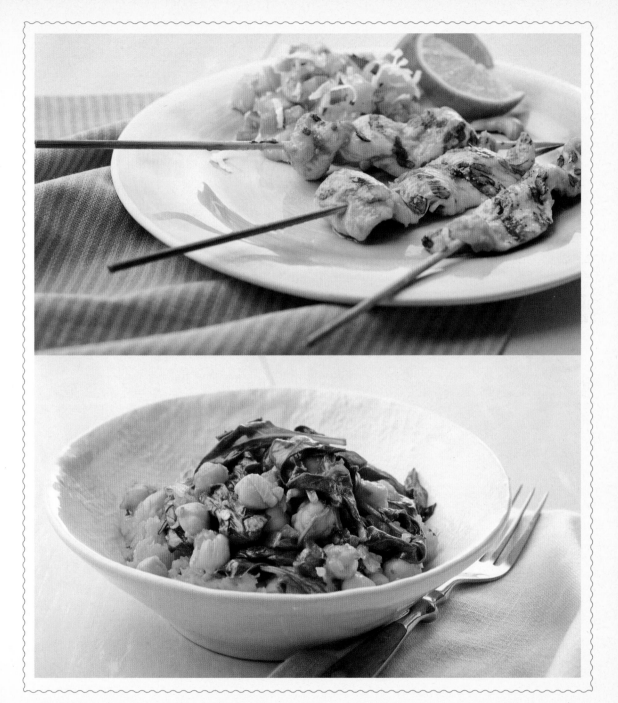

TOP: Satay, page 107, with Island Salsa, page 101 BOTTOM: Braised Coconut Spinach & Chickpeas with Lemon, page 118

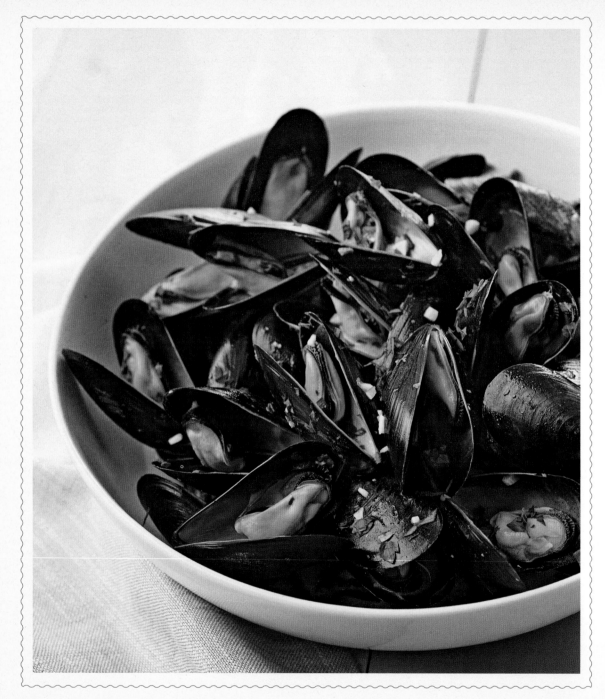

Spicy Thai Steamed Mussells, page 118

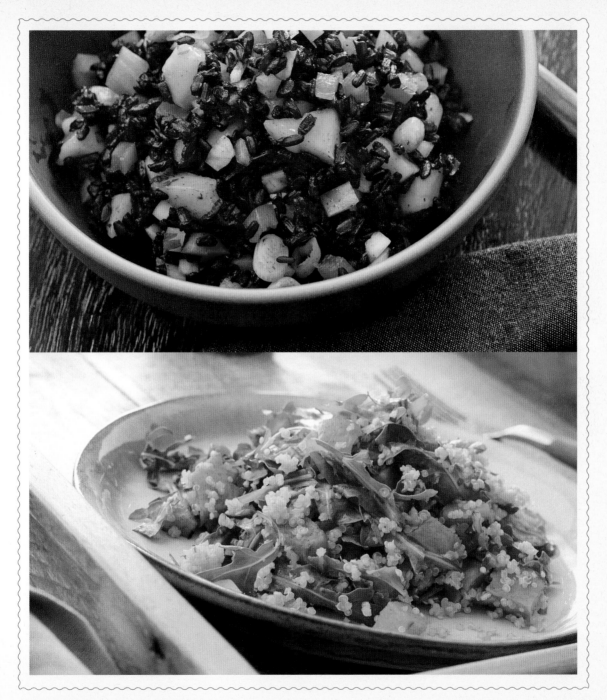

TOP: Black Rice Salad with Mango and Peanuts, page 84 BOTTOM: Roasted Sweet Potato, Quinoa, and Arugula Salad, page 89

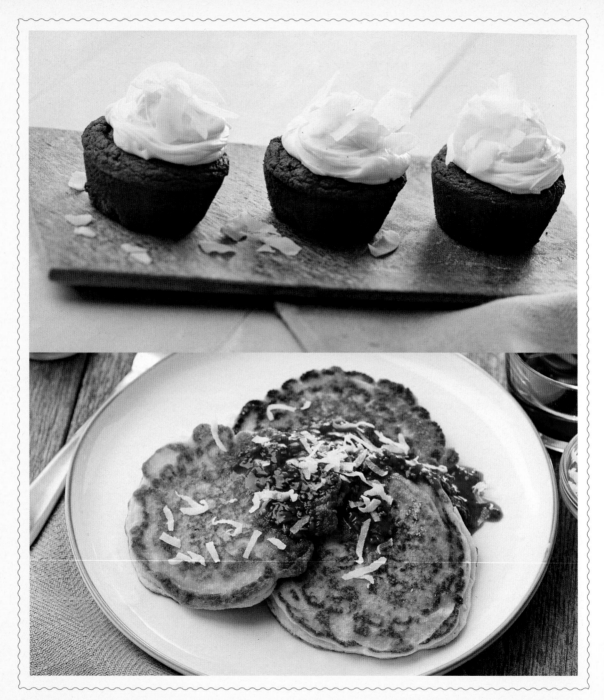

TOP: Chocoloate Coconut Cupcakes, page 131 BOTTOM: Coconut Flour Pancakes, page 69, with Red Berry Sauce, page 67

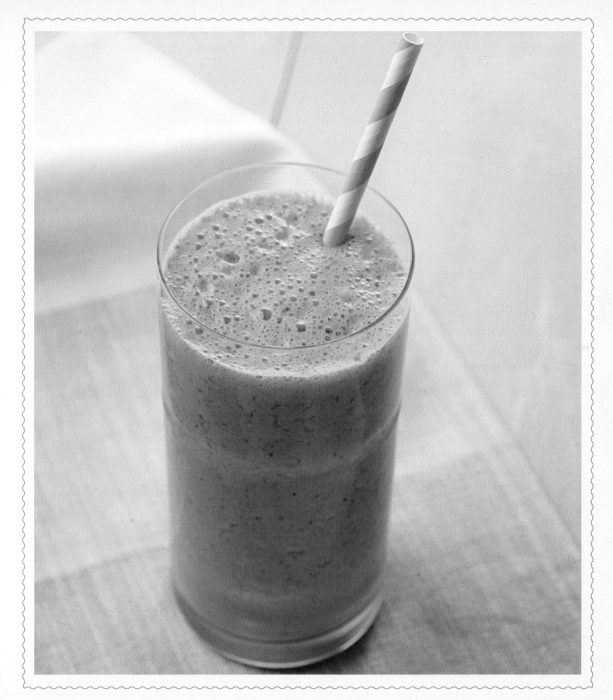

Another Green Smoothie, page 56

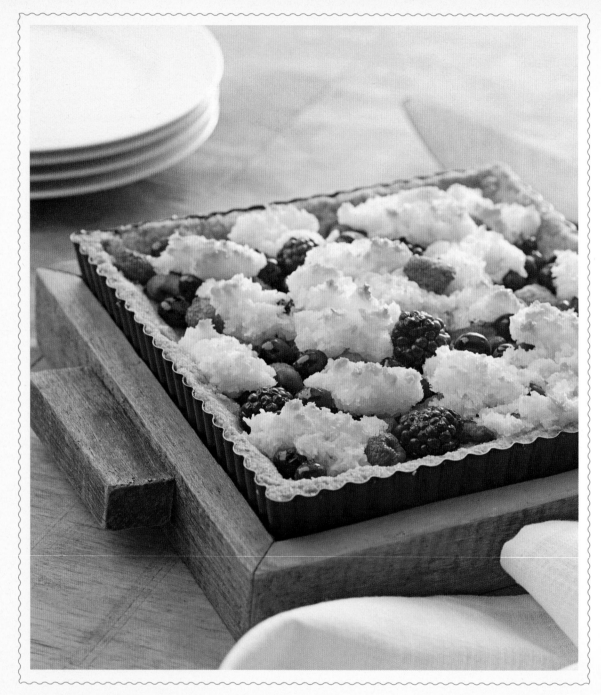

Berry Macaroon Tart, page 148

**7.** Bake the shrimp until cooked through and the coating is starting to brown, 10 to 12 minutes. Serve the shrimp with your favorite relish or salsa, such as Island Salsa on page 101.

## CRISPY COCONUT CHICKEN BITES

*MAKES 4 SERVINGS*

This healthy version of the ever-popular chicken nugget features coconut milk, coconut flour, and shredded coconut, giving you a triple dose of coconut's goodness. Serve with any of the chutneys, relishes, dips, and salsas presented in this chapter.

1 *pound chicken breasts, cut into chunks*

3 *eggs*

¼ *cup canned coconut milk*

¾ *cup coconut flour*

¾ *cup unsweetened shredded dried coconut*

¼ *teaspoon salt*

¼ *teaspoon fresh ground black pepper*

  *Coconut oil for frying*

**1.** Cut chicken breasts into "fingers," strips, or large chunks. Set aside.

**2.** In a medium bowl, beat the eggs.

**3.** Whisk coconut milk into the eggs.

**4.** In a separate shallow bowl, mix the coconut flour, shredded coconut, salt, and pepper. Stir until well combined and all lumps are gone.

**5.** While the oil is heating, start preparing the chicken: Dredge a piece of chicken in the coconut flour mix. Then, dredge it in the egg mixture, and then dredge it in the coconut flour once again. Repeat with the next piece of chicken.

**6.** Rest dredged chicken pieces on a platter, plate, or baking sheet as you finish preparing remaining chicken.

**7.** In a large frying pan, over medium heat, add ¼ to ½ inch coconut oil, enough to cover the bottom of the pan.

**8.** Reduce heat to medium-low and add a few pieces of chicken, being careful not to crowd the pan.

**9.** Fry chicken pieces on one side until golden brown, then gently turn over and cook until the other side is golden brown.

**10.** Set cooked chicken on a plate or platter that has been lined with paper towels.

**11.** Repeat with remaining chicken pieces.

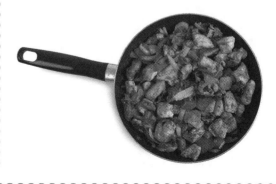

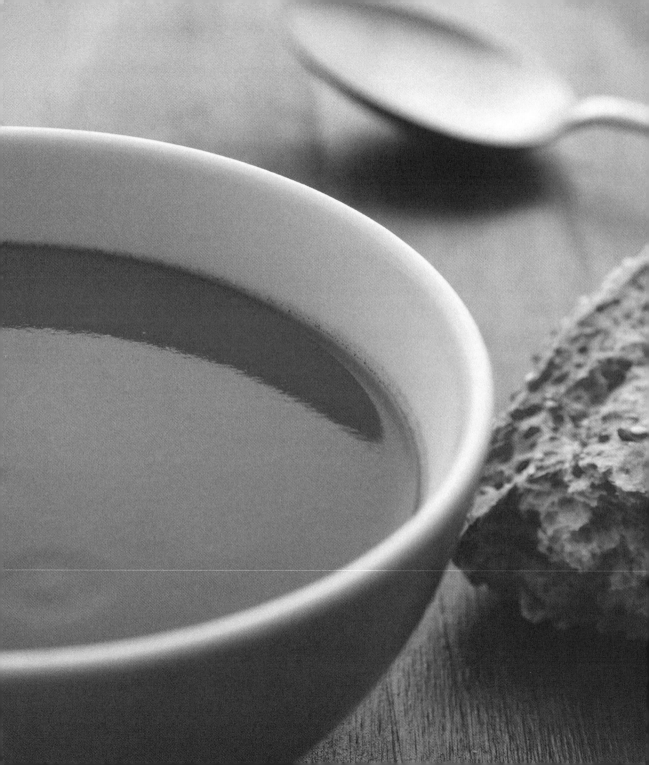

# CHAPTER 7

# COCONUT FOR DINNER

nce upon a time, dinner was really more like supper—a light meal eaten in the evening to tide you over until morning. Today, dinner is a big deal. It's when people leave their stressful work and school day behind, return home, and decompress. You know how humans use food to self-soothe? Well, dinner is often the time when we do this and eat large volumes of starchy, fatty, comforting food. In this chapter, I am going to challenge you to rethink dinner as a time to do something wonderful for yourself. The meals in this chapter are on the lighter side—I am not a fan of big dinners—and they contain coconut in its many forms, as well as other superfoods. To your health!

## SALADS

### DINNER SALAD BLUEPRINT

*MAKES 2 SERVINGS*

This is a recipe that can be played with in an infinite number of ways, so feel free to experiment and create something different at each meal!

- *3  tablespoons coconut vinegar*
- *3  tablespoons coconut aminos*
- *1½ tablespoons liquid coconut oil*
    - *Optional: 1 teaspoon coconut sugar*
    - *Optional: 1 teaspoon mustard of choice*
    - *Salt and pepper, to taste*
- *8  to 9 cups salad greens of choice*
- *1  cup chopped vegetable or mix of vegetables of choice*
- *2  to 3 cups protein (chopped chicken, beef, fish, shrimp, beans, lentils, etc.)*
    - *Optional: ½ cup chopped nuts or seeds*
    - *Optional: ¼ cup chopped fresh herbs*

**1.** In a large bowl, whisk together coconut vinegar, coconut aminos, coconut oil, coconut sugar (if desired), mustard (if desired), and salt and pepper.

**2.** Add to the bowl salad greens, chopped vegetables, protein, and if you choose to do so, nuts and/or herbs. Toss until all ingredients are coated with dressing. Serve immediately.

OPPOSITE: **Simple Tomato Soup, page 113**

## STARTER SOUPS

### BEET COCONUT SOUP

*MAKES 4 SERVINGS*

I am a beet lover. I don't think you can be a Danish-American health writer who grew up in Australia without loving beets. If you are any of these things, you'll know what I mean.

- 1 tablespoon liquid coconut oil
- 1 large onion, diced
- 3 cloves garlic, finely chopped
- 1 tablespoon finely chopped ginger
- 3 large red beets, peeled and cut into ¼-inch pieces
- 5 cups vegetable stock, divided
- 1 14-ounce can coconut milk
- ½ teaspoon salt
- ¼ teaspoon freshly ground black pepper
  Optional: chopped chives, dill, or parsley, for garnish

**1.** In a large pot, heat oil over medium heat. Sauté onion for 5 minutes.

**2.** Add garlic and ginger. Cook, stirring often, for 5 minutes.

**3.** Add beets and 4 cups of the stock. Bring to a boil, then reduce heat and simmer until beets are fork-tender, about 20 minutes.

**4.** With an immersion or regular blender, and working in batches, puree soup, adding remaining 1 cup stock, as needed, to reach desired consistency.

**5.** Stir in coconut milk, salt, and pepper.

**6.** Garnish with herbs, if desired.

### CHILLED MELON, CUCUMBER, AND COCONUT MILK SOUP

*SERVES 4 TO 6*

This unusual raw soup reminds me a bit of the koldskål (a cold Danish buttermilk soup) I grew up with—though it's much more fresh-tasting and light, thanks to the honeydew and cucumber. This would make a great starter for a vegetarian meal, or work nicely with seafood or poultry.

- 1 small honeydew melon, peeled, seeded, and cut into large chunks
- 1 medium cucumber, peeled, seeded, and cut into chunks
- ¾ cup canned coconut milk
- ¼ cup unsweetened shredded dried coconut
  Squirt of lemon or lime juice

**1.** Add all ingredients to a blender and process until absolutely smooth.

**2.** Transfer to an airtight container and refrigerate for 3 hours or overnight, until completely chilled.

## COLD-OR-NOT CARROT COCONUT SOUP

*MAKES ABOUT 6½ CUPS*

This refreshing soup can be eaten chilled, at room temperature, or warm. I prefer it warm, but it is so delicious and healthy (it contains tons of beta-carotene for great skin and eyesight) that I'll take it however I can get it.

2 *tablespoons liquid coconut oil*

1 *shallot, finely chopped*

1 *small onion, chopped*

1 *tablespoon finely grated peeled fresh gingerroot*

1 *tablespoon mild curry powder*

4 *cups chopped carrots*

2½ *cups broth*

  *Salt and pepper, to taste*

1 *to 1½ cups canned coconut milk*

1 *tablespoon fresh lime juice, plus additional to taste*

  *Water for thinning soup*

  *Optional: chopped scallions or herb of choice, for garnish*

**1.** In a large heavy saucepan, heat coconut oil over medium heat. Add shallot, onion, gingerroot, and curry powder and cook until shallot and onion are tender.

**2.** Add carrots, broth, and salt and pepper, and simmer until carrots are very tender, about 20 minutes.

**3.** With an immersion or regular blender, and working in batches, puree soup with coconut milk and lime juice until very smooth.

**4.** Adjust salt and pepper, if needed, and thin with water if necessary.

**5.** If serving warm, allow to cool to just above room temperature and ladle into soup bowls. Serve garnished with chopped scallions or herbs, if desired.

**6.** If serving soup cold, transfer soup to an airtight container and place in the refrigerator. This soup actually tastes best the second day, so I usually make it the day before and stash it in the fridge so I can garnish and serve it the next day.

## SIMPLE TOMATO SOUP

*MAKES 6 SERVINGS*

My mother couldn't cook, so most of the food we ate growing up came out of boxes, bags, and cans. Campbell's tomato soup was one of our favorites. Now that my palate is a bit more sophisticated (emphasis on "a bit"), I prefer my tomato soup homemade. If you don't like a lot spice, you can remove some or all of the ones included in this recipe, and you'll still get a beautiful bowl of soup, one that strengthens the immune system, thanks to the lycopene and vitamin C in the tomatoes, plus the antioxidant power in the spices.

4 tablespoons liquid coconut oil

2 medium yellow onions, chopped

1 teaspoon salt

3 teaspoons curry powder

1 teaspoon ground coriander

1 teaspoon ground cumin

½ teaspoon red chili pepper flakes

2 28-ounce cans whole tomatoes

4 cups chicken or vegetable broth

1 14-ounce can coconut milk

   Optional: black pepper, to taste

**1.** Add coconut oil to a large pot over medium heat. Add the onions and salt, and cook, stirring occasionally, until the onions are very soft, about 10 minutes.

**2.** Stir in the curry powder, coriander, cumin, and chili flakes, and cook, stirring constantly, about 30 seconds, or until spices are fragrant.

**3.** Add tomatoes, broth, and coconut milk and allow soup to simmer on low heat for 20 minutes.

**4.** With an immersion or regular blender, and working in batches (returning each blended batch to the warm soup pot), puree soup with coconut milk until very smooth.

**5.** Adjust seasonings and, if desired, add black pepper.

## MAIN DISHES

## SLOW COOKER COCONUT BEEF ROAST

*MAKES 4 TO 6 SERVINGS*

The slow cooker is an easy way to ensure there is always healthy food at home for you and your family to enjoy.

4 cups chicken, beef, or vegetable broth (or a mixture)

2 large onions, chopped

7 garlic cloves, minced

2 cups sliced mushrooms

1 cup chopped red pepper

½ cup sliced celery

   Salt and pepper, to taste

½ teaspoon sweet paprika

½ cup canned coconut milk (do not use "lite")

   2-pound beef rump roast

**1.** Add broth, onion, garlic, mushrooms, red pepper, celery, salt and pepper, paprika, and coconut milk to a slow cooker. Stir once.

**2.** Nestle roast among other ingredients.

**3.** Put lid on slow cooker and turn on low setting for 6 to 8 hours, or on high for 4 to 6 hours.

# CRISP COCONUT CHICKEN

*MAKES 2 SERVINGS*

This recipe uses shredded coconut instead of bread crumbs—a brilliant and delicious use of coconut! Try this dish with one or two vegetable sides for a light, nourishing dinner.

1½ cups chopped roasted red pepper
(either homemade or from a jar)

½ teaspoon fresh lemon juice

¾ teaspoon coconut sugar, divided
Pinch of cayenne

3 tablespoons liquid coconut oil, divided
Salt and pepper, to taste

1 teaspoon garlic paste (made by mashing together one medium garlic clove with ¼ teaspoon salt)

1 tablespoon Dijon-style mustard

1 whole large, skinless, boneless chicken breast (about 10 ounces), halved

½ cup gluten-free or regular all-purpose flour
Egg wash, made by whisking 1 large egg with 1 teaspoon coconut milk or water

1 cup unsweetened shredded dried coconut

**1.** Preheat oven to 375°F.

**2.** In a blender, puree the roasted red pepper with the lemon juice, ½ teaspoon of the coconut sugar, cayenne, 1 tablespoon of the coconut oil, and salt and black pepper until smooth. Set aside.

**3.** In a small bowl, whisk together the garlic paste and mustard.

**4.** Spread the garlic mixture onto both sides of the chicken. Set aside.

**5.** Get three shallow bowls ready. In one bowl, whisk together the flour, ¼ teaspoon coconut sugar, and a pinch each of salt and pepper. In the second bowl, place the egg wash. In the third, place the coconut.

**6.** Dredge the chicken in the flour, shaking off the excess.

**7.** Immediately dip the chicken into the egg wash, letting the excess drip off.

**8.** Immediately coat the chicken generously with the coconut, pressing it firmly to help the coconut adhere.

**9.** Add the remaining 2 tablespoons coconut oil to a skillet over medium-high heat. When warm, add the chicken.

**10.** Sauté chicken just until coconut is golden, about 2 minutes. Turn chicken and cook on the other side, just until coconut is golden.

**11.** Transfer chicken to a small baking dish and bake in the oven until cooked through, about 10 to 12 minutes.

**12.** Serve with red pepper sauce.

## FISH BAKED IN COCONUT MILK

*MAKES 4 SERVINGS*

This is an incredibly versatile recipe. Use salmon, tuna, or your favorite mild white fish. It all works. You will be impressed. Feel free to play with the veggies.

- 4 teaspoons lemon juice
- 2 tablespoons plus ¼ cup liquid coconut oil
  Pinch of salt
- 2 pounds thick fish fillets or steaks, halibut, cod, or salmon
- 2 cups finely chopped onion
- 2 teaspoons minced garlic
- 2 teaspoons minced ginger
- 1 teaspoon minced green serrano or jalapeño chili pepper
- 1 cup chopped tomatoes (fresh or drained canned)
- 5 teaspoons ground coriander
- 1 teaspoon ground cumin
- ¼ teaspoon cayenne powder
- ¼ teaspoon ground black pepper
- ¼ teaspoon ground turmeric
- 1 teaspoon dried parsley
- 1¼ teaspoons salt
- ½ cup canned coconut milk
- ¼ cup chopped parsley, chives, or cilantro, for garnish

**1.** Preheat oven to 350°F.

**2.** Lightly grease a baking dish large enough to hold fish in a single layer. Set aside.

**3.** Whisk together lemon juice, 2 tablespoons coconut oil, and salt in a small bowl. Set aside.

**4.** Cut fillets crosswise into 2-inch-wide strips. Rub fish with mixture of lemon juice and oil, place in the prepared baking dish, cover, and refrigerate for 1 hour.

**5.** In medium frying pan, over medium-high heat, fry onion in ¼ cup coconut oil until edges are browned.

**6.** Add garlic, ginger, and chili pepper, and stir over medium heat for 2 minutes.

**7.** Add tomatoes, coriander, cumin, cayenne powder, black pepper, turmeric, parsley, and 1¼ teaspoons salt, and fry, stirring until tomato breaks down into a chunky sauce.

**8.** Add coconut milk and simmer about 5 minutes until mixture becomes thick.

**9.** Remove fish from refrigerator, uncover, and bake for 10 minutes.

**10.** Remove fish from oven, pour sauce over fish, cover tightly with foil, and return to oven for 15 to 20 minutes or until fish is opaque.

**11.** Garnish, if desired, with chopped herbs.

# COCONUT NUT PASTA

*MAKES 4 SERVINGS*

This yummy nut pasta is made with nut butter for protein. (If you want more protein, feel free to add a cup of beans or chopped animal protein.)

1   *pound any shape pasta, regular, whole grain, or gluten-free*

2   *tablespoons liquid coconut oil*

1   *carrot, cut into matchsticks*

1   *stalk celery, sliced*

1   *cup sugar snap or snow peas, sliced on a diagonal*

½   *onion, cut into slices*

1   *cup cherry tomatoes, halved*

2   *pinches of salt*
     *Pinch of pepper*

¾   *cup canned coconut milk*

½   *cup fresh or canned diced tomatoes*

6   *tablespoons nut butter (such as almond, cashew, peanut, sunflower or other)*

2   *tablespoons ginger, finely diced*

2   *tablespoons coconut aminos or natural soy sauce (use gluten-free soy sauce if desired)*

1   *teaspoon coconut sugar or nectar*

1   *tablespoon fresh lime or lemon juice*

1   *teaspoon curry powder*

1   *teaspoon Asian chili-garlic sauce (such as sriracha)*

3   *cloves garlic, minced*

     *Optional: 1 tablespoon minced fresh parsley or cilantro*

**1.** Prepare the pasta according to package directions. Set aside.

**2.** Heat coconut oil in a large sauté pan over medium heat and add carrot, celery, peas, onion, cherry tomatoes, and 1 pinch each of salt and pepper. Sauté for 2 to 3 minutes until veggies are just barely tender. Remove pan from heat and set aside.

**3.** In a small saucepot, over medium-high heat, whisk together coconut milk, diced tomatoes, nut butter, ginger, coconut aminos, coconut sugar, lime juice, curry powder, chili-garlic sauce, garlic, minced herbs (if desired), and pinch of salt. Allow sauce to simmer for 2 to 3 minutes, whisking until smooth.

**4.** Turn off heat and add pasta and sauce to the veggies in the sauté pan. Gently toss all ingredients together. Adjust seasonings and toss to coat.

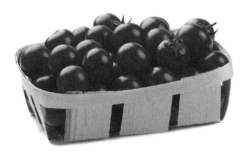

## SPICY THAI STEAMED MUSSELS

*MAKES 6 SERVINGS*

Mussels were the first nonvegetarian food I learned to make in cooking school. I couldn't believe how well they turned out. So if you've never prepared them before, give this recipe a try. You'll be pleasantly surprised. You'll also be getting an enormous amount of vitamin B12 (3 ounces of mussels contain 340 percent of the RDA for this nutrient), plus iron, calcium, magnesium, vitamins C and B6, and plenty of protein. You also get the immune system strengthening power of coconut, garlic, and curry.

5 pounds mussels (preferably cultivated)

⅓ cup lime juice

1 14-ounce can coconut milk

⅓ cup dry white wine or broth (vegetable or chicken)

1½ tablespoons Thai red curry paste

6 garlic cloves, minced

1 tablespoon Asian fish sauce

1 cup parsley or cilantro, chopped

**1.** Scrub mussels well and remove beards. Set aside.

**2.** In a large (at least 8-quart) stockpot, boil lime juice, coconut milk, wine, curry paste, garlic, and fish sauce over high heat, stirring, 2 minutes.

**3.** Add mussels, tossing to combine. Cook mussels, covered, stirring occasionally, until opened, about 5 to 8 minutes.

**4.** Discard any unopened mussels.

**5.** Toss herbs with mussels.

## BRAISED COCONUT SPINACH & CHICKPEAS WITH LEMON

*MAKES 4 SERVINGS*

Tender braised greens and chickpeas create a beautiful ragout-like dish that is lovely served over pureed sweet potatoes, brown rice, millet, quinoa, polenta, potatoes, mashed cauliflower, or anything else. Your taste buds will thank you. So will your body: This dish is high in vitamins A, C, and E, as well as protein, zinc, magnesium, and fiber.

2 tablespoons liquid coconut oil

1 small yellow onion, diced

5 to 6 garlic cloves, minced

1 tablespoon grated fresh ginger

¼ to ½ teaspoon red pepper flakes

1 15-ounce can chickpeas, drained

1 pound baby spinach

1 14-ounce can coconut milk

2 tablespoons lemon juice

¼ cup tomato paste

1 teaspoon salt, or to taste

Pepper, to taste

**1.** Heat the coconut oil in a large saucepan over medium-high heat. Add the onion and cook for about 5 minutes, or until it begins to brown.

**2.** Add the garlic, ginger, and red pepper. Cook for 3 minutes, stirring frequently.

**3.** Add chickpeas and cook over high heat for 2 minutes or until the chickpeas are beginning to turn golden.

**4.** Add spinach, in batches if needed.

**5.** Add coconut milk, lemon juice, tomato paste, and salt and pepper. Bring to a simmer, then turn down the heat and cook for 10 minutes, or until the chickpeas are warmed through.

**6.** Adjust seasoning before serving.

## COCONUT MASHED POTATOES

*MAKES 4 TO 6 SERVINGS*

You mashed potato lovers will be thrilled to know that you can have your favorite food and get the coconut your body so deeply desires—all in this simple dish. Feel free to add 1 or 2 cups of finely chopped cooked greens to the mashies and enjoy!

2   *pounds russet or Yukon Gold potatoes*

1   *cup canned coconut milk*
    *Salt and pepper, to taste*

¼   *cup liquid coconut oil*

**1.** Add salted water to a large pot over high heat and boil potatoes until soft but not falling apart.

**2.** Drain potatoes in a colander and return to pot.

**3.** Add coconut milk and salt and pepper. Using a potato masher, mash potatoes until chunky.

**4.** Add coconut oil and continue mashing until smooth. Adjust seasoning.

## HEARTY SIDES

## COCONUT SCALLOPED POTATOES

*MAKES 6 SERVINGS*

Traditional scalloped potatoes really aren't that good for you. Fortunately, there is an alternative—this delicious scalloped potato recipe, which celebrates the considerable benefits of coconut milk. You will love it!

*Coconut oil for greasing dish*

1   *14-ounce can coconut milk*

2   *cups vegetable or chicken broth*

1½  *teaspoons salt*

½   *teaspoon dried thyme*

1   *pound russet or Yukon Gold potatoes, peeled, cut crosswise or lengthwise (depending on their size) into ¼-inch-thick slices, and submerged in a bowl of cold water to prevent browning*

6   *scallions (green tops and white bulbs), thinly sliced crosswise*

**1.** Preheat oven to 350°F.

**2.** Lightly grease a 2½- to 3-quart casserole dish with coconut oil. Set aside.

**3.** In a small bowl, whisk together coconut milk, broth, salt, and thyme.

**4.** Drain the potatoes and pat dry with a paper towel or clean dishcloth.

**5.** Cover the bottom of the casserole dish with a layer of potatoes, and sprinkle with ⅓ of the scallions.

**6.** Stir the coconut milk mixture and drizzle ⅓ of it over the potatoes and scallions.

**7.** Repeat the layers of potatoes, scallions, and coconut milk mixture 2 more times, ending with a layer of potatoes, scallions and coconut milk mixture.

**8.** Cover and bake for 30 to 45 minutes, until potatoes are just tender.

**9.** Remove the cover and continue to bake until the potatoes are browned, 10 to 15 minutes. Then serve.

## VEGETABLE MILLET PILAF

*MAKES 4 SERVINGS*

Millet is actually a seed—one that is high in fiber, protein, iron, magnesium, manganese, zinc, omega-3 fatty acids, amino acids, and lignans (which protect against cancer and heart disease, and help heal digestive disorders).

1   tablespoon liquid coconut oil

1   shallot or ½ medium onion, minced

4   cloves garlic, chopped

1   cup uncooked millet

1   medium zucchini or yellow squash, diced

½   cup sliced baby bella mushrooms

1   cup vegetable or chicken broth

1   cup canned coconut milk

     Salt and pepper, to taste

**1.** Heat coconut oil in a medium saucepan over medium-high heat. Add the shallot and cook for 2 or 3 minutes until it begins to soften.

**2.** Add garlic and the millet and stir to coat. Let the millet toast for 1 or 2 minutes.

**3.** Add the zucchini and mushrooms and sauté for 2 to 3 minutes.

**4.** Add the broth and coconut milk and let the liquid come to a boil. Turn down the heat to medium-low and cover. Check every 5 minutes or so but don't stir.

**5.** Once all of the liquid is absorbed, take the millet off heat and allow it to sit for 5 minutes with the cover on.

**6.** Fluff the millet with a fork and add salt and pepper to taste.

## COCONUT BROWN RICE

*MAKES 6 SERVINGS*

Coconut rice is one of my kids' favorite side dishes. It is full of fiber and protein, and boasts an incredible array of minerals (manganese, selenium, magnesium). Coconut Brown Rice is the perfect foil for curries, sautés, stir-fry, and other saucy dishes. It's also a great base for more elaborate dishes: Just add nuts, dried fruit, beans, or other ingredients and you've got yourself a pilaf.

> 2½ cups water
>
> 1  14-ounce can coconut milk
>
> ½  teaspoon salt
>
> 2  cups brown rice

**1.** In a medium saucepot, bring water, coconut milk, and salt to a boil.

**2.** Add rice, stir just once, reduce heat to low, and cover.

**3.** Simmer for about 45 minutes (without stirring even once—that's what makes rice mushy!) or until rice is cooked and grains are separated and fluffy with no liquid left in the pot. You can lift the lid once or twice while rice cooks to check on it, but quickly replace the lid.

## CAULIFLOWER MASHED "POTATOES"

*MAKES 6 SERVINGS*

This is an absolutely delicious, as well as a sneaky, way to get high levels of vitamins C and K, manganese, and anti-inflammatory phytonutrients into your diet. And did I mention how delicious it is?

> 5  cups roughly chopped cauliflower
>
> 5  cloves garlic
>
> 1  cup canned coconut milk
>
> 2  tablespoons liquid coconut oil
>
> 1  teaspoon salt
>
> 1  teaspoon black pepper
>
> Optional: 2 tablespoons chopped chives or parsley

**1.** Fill a large pot with salted water and bring to a boil. Add cauliflower and garlic cloves and simmer over low heat for 8 minutes or until soft but not mushy.

**2.** Drain cauliflower and garlic and place in a food processor. Pulse until chunky.

**3.** Add coconut milk, coconut oil, and salt and pepper, and pulse until smooth.

**4.** Transfer to a serving dish and, if desired, garnish with chopped herbs.

## VEGGIE SIDES

### COCONUT MILK–BRAISED GREENS

*MAKES 4 SERVINGS*

Feel free to add chopped nuts, shredded dried coconut, or even raisins to the finished dish. Delicious.

- 1  pound (about 2 bunches) collard greens, kale, or mustard greens, stems and ribs removed, roughly chopped
- 2  tablespoons liquid coconut oil
- 1  small yellow onion, thinly sliced
- ¾  cup canned coconut milk
- 1  tablespoon lemon juice
   Salt, to taste
   Black pepper, to taste

**1.** Bring a large pot of salted water to a boil. Add greens and cook for 2 minutes. Drain well in a colander and set aside.

**2.** Heat coconut oil in a large skillet over medium heat. Add onions and cook about 5 minutes, stirring often, until onions are tender and translucent.

**3.** Add greens, coconut milk, and lemon juice to the skillet. Stir and allow to simmer until tender, about 7 minutes.

**4.** Season with salt and pepper.

### SOUTHEAST ASIAN BROCCOLI

*MAKES 2 SERVINGS*

One of the first foods to be named a "superfood," broccoli contains high levels of vitamin K, vitamin C, vitamin B6, vitamin E, vitamin B2, vitamin A, and vitamin B1, as well as chromium, folate, fiber, pantothenic acid, manganese, choline, potassium, and a mix of cancer-fighting phytonutrients.

- 1  tablespoon liquid coconut oil
- 2  heads broccoli, including the upper part of the stalk, chopped into dice-size pieces
   Salt, to taste
- 5  tablespoons canned coconut milk, divided
- 2  scallions, thinly sliced
- 1  large lime, zested and juiced
- 1  clove garlic, minced
- 1  small piece ginger, minced
- ¼  teaspoon ground coriander
- ¼  teaspoon ground red chili pepper
   Optional garnish: 1 tablespoon unsweetened dried shredded coconut

**1.** Heat coconut oil in a large skillet over medium-high heat.

**2.** When the oil is hot, add the broccoli and some salt. Stir-fry the broccoli for a minute.

**3.** Add 2 tablespoons of the coconut milk to the broccoli and cook just until broccoli begins to get tender-crisp.

**4.** Remove broccoli from heat and stir in the scallions, lime zest and juice, garlic, ginger, spices, and remaining coconut milk. Adjust salt if necessary. Toss to combine.

**5.** Garnish with shredded dried coconut, if desired.

## SHREDDED SUMMER SQUASH

*MAKES 2 SERVINGS*

This is how zucchini is done in the Pedersen household. (We often tuck it into burritos or pasta.)

1   *tablespoon liquid coconut oil*

1   *garlic clove, minced*

6   *small or 4 medium zucchini or yellow crookneck squash, shredded on a box grater*
    *Salt and pepper, to taste*

2   *tablespoons canned coconut milk*
    *Optional: 1 tablespoon minced herb or herbs of choice*

**1.** Heat coconut oil in a large skillet over medium heat. Add garlic and cook for 30 seconds.

**2.** Add shredded squash to skillet. Season with salt and pepper and add coconut milk. Cook for 2 to 5 minutes, until just tender and liquid has mostly evaporated.

**3.** Garnish with herbs, if desired.

## ROASTED VEGGIES IN COCONUT OIL

*MAKES 8 SERVINGS*

Play with this recipe—you can use equal amounts of radish, rutabaga, fennel, burdock, kohlrabi, broccoli stems, Brussels sprouts, or anything else that strikes your fancy! No matter which veggie you roast, it will be a revelation.

4   *to 5 carrots, peeled*

2   *medium onions, peeled*

1   *acorn squash, cleaned and peeled*

1   *large sweet potato, peeled*

3   *to 4 small red potatoes*

1   *medium beet, peeled*

¼   *cup coconut oil*
    *Unrefined sea salt, to taste*
    *Freshly ground black pepper, to taste*
    *Optional: 1 or more tablespoons fresh chopped herb, such as thyme*

**1.** Preheat oven to 425°F.

**2.** Cut all vegetables into similarly sized pieces.

**3.** Place vegetables in a bowl, drizzle with coconut oil, and sprinkle with salt and pepper and optional herb. Using clean hands, toss veggies until all are coated.

**4.** Place vegetables in a single layer on 1 or 2 rimless baking sheets.

**5.** Roast for 25 to 35 minutes or until all the vegetables are tender, turning once.

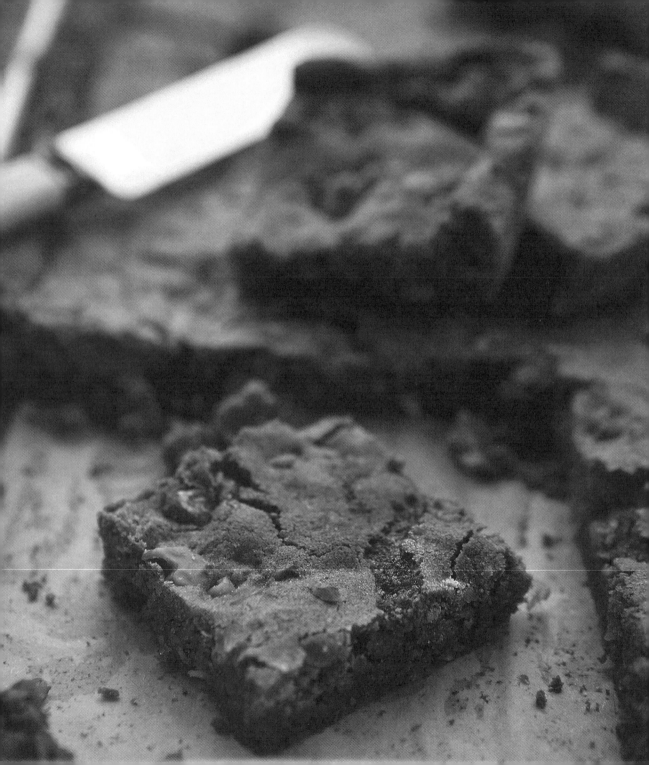

# CHAPTER 8

# COCONUT DESSERTS AND OTHER SWEETS

As much as it pains the nutritionist in me to admit this, coconut is the quintessential dessert ingredient. Say the word "coconut" and most people aren't even going to consider coconut water, coconut flour, or coconut oil. What they'll think of, instead, is chocolate-covered coconut candy bars, coconut cake, creamy pies, coconut shortbread, and various other sweet confections—all of which makes including a dessert chapter in this book a natural addition.

But—and this is a big "but"—unlike mainstream coconut sweets, the ones in this chapter are actually good for you. The recipes are filled with coconut in all its magnificence. Here, you'll find delectable coconut bars, coconut cakes, coconut cookies, coconut candy, and dozens of other goodies—all of which have been developed to delight your taste buds as well as nourish your body.

## BARS

### APRICOT COCONUT BARS

*MAKES 9 BARS*

As a child in Australia, one of my favorite treats was a dried apricot–coconut candy bar. It remains the closest thing to heaven I've ever tasted. I rarely get back to Oz for those bars—but this homemade version makes me just as happy. It is rich in fiber, protein, vitamins, and minerals, and it's my favorite nutrient-dense pick-me-up.

- *½ cup unsalted cashews*
- *1 cup dried apricots*
- *¾ cup unsweetened shredded dried coconut*
- *⅓ cup rolled oats*
- *2 tablespoons coconut nectar or honey*
- *1 tablespoon liquid coconut oil*
- *2 tablespoons hempseed*
- *¼ teaspoon sea salt*

**1.** Line an 8-by-8-inch baking pan with foil or parchment paper. Set aside.

**2.** In a food processor, pulse cashews just until coarsely chopped. Empty these into a small bowl and set aside.

OPPOSITE: **Brownies Extraordinaire, page 127**

**3.** Pulse apricots in a food processor until finely chopped. Add coconut, oats, coconut nectar, coconut oil, hempseed, and salt, pulsing until well combined.

**4.** Add chopped cashews to the mixture and pulse a couple of times until combined.

**5.** Firmly press mixture into prepared pan. Smooth surface.

**6.** Place pan in the freezer for 1 or 2 hours.

**7.** Using a wet knife, cut into bars.

**8.** Store uneaten bars in the refrigerator.

---

### COCONUT FLOUR RECIPES: WHAT'S WITH ALL THE EGGS?

If you've ever baked with coconut flour—or even if you've ever looked up coconut recipes in your favorite healthy cookbook or online—you've probably noticed that most recipes contain a large number of eggs. There's a reason for that: Coconut flour is an absorbent flour, and one that does not bind together well. Eggs give coconut flour-based recipes a moister consistency and help these goodies stick together so they are not a dry, clumpy mess of crumbs! When baking with coconut flour, you usually want to use about 3 or more eggs (or the equivalent egg replacement) for every ½ cup of flour.

---

## COCONUT CRISPIES

*MAKES 9 BARS*

I grew up eating Rice Krispies Treats made with melted margarine and marshmallows. I still love the idea of those classic sweets, but I feed my children this healthier superfood version. Keep Coconut Crispies in the freezer or fridge so they stay firm.

*¼ cup organic thick (not runny) almond, cashew, peanut, sunflower, or other nut butter*

*¼ cup coconut oil*

*1½ tablespoons coconut nectar*

  *Pinch of salt*

  *Optional: 1½ teaspoons organic vanilla*

  *Optional: 1½ teaspoons organic cinnamon or pumpkin pie spice*

*2 cups brown rice cereal (you can also used puffed quinoa, millet, or barley cereal)*

*1 cup finely shredded unsweetened dried coconut*

**1.** Line an 8-by-8-inch baking pan with foil.

**2.** In a large saucepan over low heat, melt together nut butter and coconut oil.

**3.** Whisk in coconut nectar, pinch of salt, and if desired, vanilla and spice. Keep stirring until mixture is smooth.

**4.** Add cereal and shredded coconut, stirring until thoroughly coated.

**5.** Firmly press mixture into prepared pan.

**6.** Place pan in freezer for 2 hours or overnight.

**7.** Using a sharp knife, slice into 9 bars.

**8.** Store uneaten treats in refrigerator.

## BROWNIES EXTRAORDINAIRE

*MAKES ABOUT 9 BROWNIES*

If you are like me, you've spent years searching for the best brownie recipe. This one may be it. It has a very faint coconut taste that beautifully complements the full-on chocolaty goodness. Plus, you get the brain, heart, skin, and immune system benefits of coconut flour, coconut oil, and coconut milk. Last, these brownies are gluten- and grain-free, making them great for you if you have celiac disease or are on a Paleo diet.

*½ cup coconut flour*

*½ cup unsweetened cocoa powder*

*½ teaspoon salt*

*½ teaspoon baking soda*

> *Optional: ¼ teaspoon allspice or cinnamon or pumpkin pie spice*

*5 large eggs*

*⅓ cup liquid coconut oil*

*¾ cup coconut nectar (or Grade B maple syrup, honey, or a blend of the two)*

*1 teaspoon vanilla extract*

*2 tablespoons canned coconut milk (do not use "lite")*

**1.** Preheat oven to 350°F.

**2.** Lightly grease an 8-by-8-inch baking pan. Set aside.

**3.** In a large bowl, whisk together coconut flour, cocoa powder, salt, baking soda, and allspice (if desired) until thoroughly combined and clump-free. Set aside.

**4.** Using a stand mixer with a paddle attachment, blend together eggs, coconut oil, coconut nectar, vanilla extract, and coconut milk on a low speed. Continue until thoroughly combined.

**5.** Add the coconut flour mixture to the egg mixture and blend on a low speed until well combined.

**6.** Pour batter into prepared pan.

**7.** Bake for 25 minutes or until a toothpick inserted in the middle comes out clean.

**8.** Allow brownies to cool before cutting into bars with a wet knife.

### MAKE YOUR OWN ALMOND FLOUR

If you don't have almond flour on hand—and need it for a recipe—don't panic. It's easy to make your own! Simply place whole or sliced, raw or roasted almonds in a food processor and pulse until the nuts are pulverized. Be careful not to overprocess the almonds, however—otherwise you'll end up with almond butter.

# PUMPKIN PIE BARS

*MAKES 9 BARS*

I love pumpkin and coconut together—which is why these scrumptious bars are one of my favorites. They are rich in beta-carotene, fiber, protein, minerals, phytonutrients, and omega-3 fatty acids.

- ½ cup old-fashioned rolled oats (certified gluten-free if necessary)
- ½ cup pumpkin seeds
- ½ cup unsweetened shredded dried coconut
- ½ teaspoon cinnamon
- ⅜ teaspoon salt, divided
- ⅔ cup pitted dates, chopped (plus a few more if needed)
- 1½ cups pumpkin puree
- ⅓ cup coconut nectar or Grade B maple syrup
- ¼ cup liquid coconut oil
- 1 teaspoon vanilla
- 2 teaspoons pumpkin pie spice (or any blend of cinnamon, ginger, cloves, allspice, and/or cardamom)
- ⅛ teaspoon black pepper
- 2 tablespoons coconut flour

**1.** Line an 8-by-8-inch baking pan with foil or parchment paper so you'll easily be able to lift the bars out of the pan and cut them.

**2.** To make the crust: Place the oats, pumpkin seeds, shredded coconut, cinnamon, and ⅛ teaspoon of the salt in a food processor. Pulse just until finely ground.

**3.** Add ⅔ cup dates and process until well combined and sticky. The mixture may look crumbly, but it should hold together when pinched between your fingers. If necessary, add more dates to get the right consistency.

## HOW TO "HEALTHY UP" A BOXED CAKE MIX

When I was growing up, most families made cakes from store-bought mixes that came in a box. These mixes may have been convenient and certainly delivered foolproof results in a jiffy, but they were—and still are—chock-full of chemical ingredients that are not so good for you. For a more nutritious alternative, head over to your local health food store and check out some of the whole-food cake mixes that are made by companies like Bob's Red Mill and Arrowhead Mills. To make these mixes even healthier, just replace the oil or melted butter that may be called for with liquid coconut oil. You can also use coconut milk to replace any liquids. These are easy, delicious ways to add omega-3 fatty acids, brain-supporting lauric acid, and cardiovascular heart-protective medium chain fatty acids to your baked goods.

**4.** Press the dough firmly and evenly into the baking pan. Place the pan in the freezer.

**5.** To make the filling: Combine the pumpkin puree, coconut nectar, coconut oil, vanilla, ¼ teaspoon salt, pumpkin pie spice, and black pepper in a food processor. Blend until smooth.

**6.** Add the coconut flour and blend until well combined.

**7.** Remove the pan from the freezer and pour the filling on top, spreading it out evenly. Cover and refrigerate for at least 6 hours or overnight.

**8.** Lift the bars out of the pan using the edges of the foil or parchment paper. Use a wet chef's knife to cut bars, wiping the knife clean between cuts. Serve chilled.

**9.** Store uneaten bars in refrigerator.

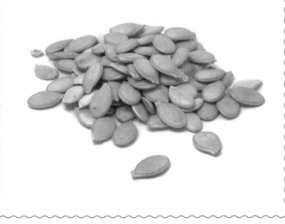

# PURE COCONUT BARS

*MAKES 9 BARS*

This fun recipe is pure coconut—and it's filled with fats that are healthy for your brain, fiber, protein, antioxidants, and phytonutrients. Chocolate lovers may want to add ½ cup chopped dark raw chocolate to the mix—or add chopped macadamia nuts, cashews, or almonds, if you like.

> 2 *cups unsweetened shredded dried coconut*
>
> ⅓ *cup coconut nectar or Grade B maple syrup*
>
> 4 *tablespoons liquid coconut oil*
>
> 1 *teaspoon pure vanilla extract*
>
> ¼ *teaspoon salt*

**1.** Line an 8-by-8-inch baking pan with foil. Set aside.

**2.** Combine all ingredients in a food processor. Pulse until ingredients are well combined and mixture is smooth.

**3.** Firmly press mixture into prepared pan, smoothing the top.

**4.** Allow the mixture to set in the freezer for 1 hour or in the refrigerator for 3 hours before serving.

**5.** Cut bars with a wet knife.

## CUPS AND CAKES

### ALMOND-COCONUT POUND CAKE

*MAKES 8 SERVINGS*

Dense, flavorful, and rich with protein, vitamins, fiber, and antioxidants, this wonderful cake is a healthier, better-tasting (in my opinion!) twist on the traditional pound cake. Sometimes I dress it up even more by adding chunks of almond paste or marzipan to the batter. I've even slipped in chopped dark chocolate, though my favorite way to enjoy this recipe is just as it's written. Because this cake contains so much almond flour, it is a bit pricey to make, so save it for someone who loves almonds.

- 3   cups almond flour
- ¼   cup coconut flour
- ¾   teaspoon baking soda
- 1   teaspoon baking powder
- ½   teaspoon salt
- ½   cup liquid coconut oil
- ⅔   cup coconut sugar
- 4   large eggs
- ½   cup canned coconut milk
- ½   teaspoon almond extract
- 1   teaspoon vanilla extract

**1.** Preheat oven to 350°F.

**2.** Grease a mini loaf pan with a light coating of coconut oil.

**3.** In a large bowl, whisk together almond flour, coconut flour, baking soda, baking powder, and salt.

**4.** In the bowl of a stand mixer, blend together liquid coconut oil, coconut sugar, eggs, coconut milk, almond extract, and vanilla extract on a medium speed.

**5.** Add dry ingredients to liquid mixture 1 cup at a time, blending between additions. Blend just until smooth.

**6.** Scrape batter into prepared pan, smoothing the top.

**7.** Bake for 35 to 45 minutes, or until a cake tester inserted in the middle of the cake comes out clean.

**8.** Allow cake to cool for 15 minutes before slicing.

### GLUTEN-FREE FUDGE CAKE

*MAKES 4 SERVINGS*

Rich, chocolaty, and gluten-free, this fudge cake is baked in individual portions. Coconut flour, coconut oil, and coconut sugar create a moist, nutrient-dense cake. This outrageous dessert is best tackled by more experienced bakers.

⅔ cup dark or semisweet chocolate chips
(or 4.2 ounces of chocolate)

4 tablespoons liquid coconut oil

2 large eggs

1 teaspoon vanilla extract

⅛ teaspoon salt

2 tablespoons coconut sugar

1 teaspoon coconut flour

2 teaspoons cocoa powder

**1.** Preheat oven to 375°F.

**2.** Grease and flour four 6-ounce ramekins using coconut oil and coconut flour or another gluten-free flour. Place them on a baking sheet.

**3.** In a double boiler or a saucepan over very low heat, melt chocolate with the coconut oil. Set aside.

**4.** In the bowl of a stand mixer, using the paddle attachment, beat together eggs, vanilla, salt, and coconut sugar until frothy, about 4 to 5 minutes on medium-low setting.

**5.** Slowly mix in melted chocolate and coconut oil.

**6.** Gently add in coconut flour and cocoa powder. Keep mixing until batter is smooth.

**7.** Pour batter evenly into ramekins.

**8.** Bake for 10 to 13 minutes.

# CHOCOLATE COCONUT CUPCAKES

*MAKES 12 CUPCAKES*

Yum!!! You will love these gluten-free cupcakes! They are packed with all the goodness of coconut, including lauric acid, protein, fiber, and phytonutrients for healthy nervous system and immune system function. (Note that the batter is very thin.) If you're using purchased applesauce or pumpkin puree, check the ingredients. These are not gluten-containing foods, but you never know what some food companies add to their products!

1⅔ cups gluten-free baking flour

⅓ cup coconut flour

2 teaspoons baking soda

1 teaspoon baking powder
Pinch of salt

¾ cup cocoa

1 cup hot water or coffee

1 cup water or orange juice

4 large eggs

½ cup liquid coconut oil

½ cup applesauce, mashed banana,
or pumpkin puree

1 cup coconut sugar

1 cup canned coconut milk
Optional: gluten-free frosting or topping of choice
Optional: ¼ cup shredded dried coconut for garnish

**1.** Preheat oven to 350°F.

**2.** Lightly grease a 12-cup muffin tin with coconut oil (or use paper cupcake liners).

**3.** In a large bowl, whisk together the flours, baking soda, baking powder, and salt. Set aside.

**4.** In a second bowl, mix the cocoa with the hot water or coffee. Stir in the additional cup of water or orange juice. Set aside.

**5.** In the bowl of a stand mixer, cream together the eggs, coconut oil, applesauce, coconut sugar, and coconut milk.

**6.** To the creamed egg-applesauce mixture, add ⅓ of the flour mixture. Blend until combined, then add ⅓ of the cocoa-liquid mixture. Blend. Repeat 2 more times until everything is blended into a smooth batter.

**7.** Pour the batter into the prepared muffin cups until each is almost ¾ full.

**8.** Bake for 20 minutes, or until a toothpick in the center comes out clean.

**9.** If you like, frost cupcakes once they have thoroughly cooled.

**10.** For a dramatic presentation, scatter some shredded coconut over the frosting.

## MAKING YOUR OWN SWEETENED SHREDDED COCONUT

To make a healthier version of sweetened flake coconut, put 2 cups of unsweetened shredded dried coconut in a large zip storage bag or a storage container. Add in 1 or 2 tablespoons of coconut sugar that you have pulverized into powder using a coffee grinder, food processor, or high-power blender (such as a Vitamix or Blendtec). Store in a cool location. Shake or stir well before using.

# GINGER-LIME COCONUT POUND CAKE

*MAKES 8 SERVINGS*

This is another dense, moist pound cake. I love it made only with lime, only with ginger, and with both flavors together. Try making this pound cake all 3 ways and find your favorite! No matter how you flavor it, you're getting a hefty dose of lauric acid to help promote stable moods and brain health, and medium chain fatty acids to keep your cardiovascular system at its strongest.

**Cake**

1⅓ cup unbleached all-purpose flour
    (regular or gluten-free)

⅓  cup coconut flour

2  teaspoons baking powder

¼ teaspoon salt

½ cup coconut oil

¼ cup coconut sugar

4 large eggs

½ cup canned coconut milk (do not use "lite")

2 teaspoons vanilla extract

2 tablespoons lime zest

¼ tablespoon lime juice

1 tablespoon fresh ginger, minced or grated

¼ cup unsweetened shredded dried coconut

¼ cup crystallized ginger, chopped fine

**Glaze**

¼ cup coconut sugar

¼ cup lime juice

**1.** Preheat oven to 350°F.

**2.** Lightly grease a 4-by-8-inch loaf pan with coconut oil.

**3.** In a large bowl, whisk together both flours, baking powder, and salt. Set aside.

**4.** In a large bowl of a standing mixer, cream the coconut oil with ¼ cup coconut sugar. The mixture will appear crumbly.

**5.** Add the eggs, one at a time, beating well between each addition. The mixture will become creamy-looking.

**6.** To the mixer bowl, add coconut milk, vanilla, lime zest, ¼ tablespoon lime juice, and fresh ginger. Beat once more.

**7.** Add the flour mixture to the batter and mix only until just combined. Do not overmix.

**8.** Gently stir in dried coconut and crystallized ginger.

**9.** Pour the batter into prepared loaf pan.

**10.** Bake for 45 minutes, or until a toothpick inserted into the center comes out clean.

**11.** While the cake bakes, make the glaze: Whisk together ¼ cup coconut sugar with ¼ cup lime juice in a small saucepan over medium-low heat. Simmer until sugar is completely dissolved, about 1 minute.

**12.** Immediately upon removing the cake from the oven, poke holes in it using a toothpick or thin skewer. Using a pastry brush, brush glaze over the cake. Or use a spoon and smooth glaze over the top of the cake.

**13.** Allow cake to cool completely before slicing.

---

### EASY COCONUT FROSTING

In a large bowl of a stand mixer, add ½ cup coconut butter, 1 teaspoon vanilla extract, and 2 tablespoons coconut nectar. (You can add 1 teaspoon of cocoa powder to make chocolate frosting.) Using a whisk attachment, beat on a high speed until blended and light and fluffy. This makes enough to frost 6 to 12 cupcakes.

## DARK BARK

*MAKES 4 SERVINGS*

This recipe is easy, fun, and customizable.

- 1  *cup coconut sugar*
- 1  *cup cocoa*
- 1½ *cups unsweetened shredded dried coconut*
- 1½ *cups liquid coconut oil*
-    *Pinch of salt*
- ¼  *cup coarsely or finely chopped nuts or seeds*
- ¼  *cup dried fruit, chopped if large*

**1.** In a food processor, pulse coconut sugar until powdery.

**2.** Add cocoa and shredded coconut and pulse 2 or 3 times just to blend.

**3.** In a large bowl, whisk together the blended coconut-cocoa mixture with the coconut oil and salt. Mix until smooth.

**4.** Stir in chopped nuts and fruit.

**5.** Using a spatula, scrape chocolate mixture onto wax paper or a nonstick baking mat, spreading mixture to about ¼ inch in height.

**6.** Move wax paper or nonstick baking mat with the chocolate to the fridge and chill for 45 minutes or more.

**7.** Break bark into pieces (you get to choose the size).

**8.** Store uneaten candy in a sealed container in the refrigerator.

## CANDY

## APRICOT BITES

*MAKES 8 PIECES*

I promise that even if you don't love apricots as much as I do, you'll love this sprightly, addictive treat. The apricots are rich in beta-carotene, for a healthy immune system, eyes, and skin. There are generous amounts of fiber in the apricots and coconut, plus the coconut butter and coconut oil provide medium chain fatty acids for cardiovascular health.

- 1  *cup dried apricots, divided*
- ⅓  *cup unsweetened shredded dried coconut*
- 5  *tablespoons coconut butter*
- 2  *tablespoons coconut oil*
-    *Zest of 1 lemon or lime*

**1.** Lightly grease a mini (5½-by-3-by-2½-inch) loaf pan with coconut oil, or line the pan with wax paper. Set aside.

**2.** Add ½ cup of the dried apricots to the bowl of a food processor. Pulse until the apricots are chopped into medium pieces. Remove to a large bowl and set aside.

**3.** In the same food processor bowl, add the remaining ½ cup dried apricots and process into a creamy paste.

**4.** Add apricot paste and remaining ingredients to the chopped apricots. Mix together, by hand, until ingredients are thoroughly combined.

**5.** Scrape batter into prepared pan, smoothing the top.

**6.** Refrigerate for 1 hour or more until firm. Cut into small squares.

## WHITE FUDGE

*MAKES 12 PIECES*

Did you know this fudge could, potentially, help keep colds, flu, and other viruses at bay? Well, that hasn't exactly been proven, but coconut oil and coconut butter have been proven to have antiviral, antibacterial, antifungal, and even antiparasitic healing properties. Research has also shown that coconut oil and the coconut flesh in coconut butter help support overall immune system functions. The cashews add protein and fiber to this fudge. And did I mention how delicious this dessert is?

- *1 cup cashews*
- *1 cup coconut butter*
- *½ cup cocoa butter*
- *¼ cup coconut nectar or Grade B maple syrup*
- *1 teaspoon vanilla extract*
- *¼ teaspoon salt*

**1.** Lightly grease a mini-muffin pan or fill the cups with muffin liners. If you have chocolate molds, you can use them instead of a mini-muffin pan. Set aside.

**2.** In a food processor or high-speed blender, blend cashews into a paste.

**3.** In a saucepan over medium heat, combine pureed cashews with remaining ingredients. Stir often until ingredients are combined and warmed through, about 5 minutes.

**4.** Spoon cooked fudge mixture into prepared muffin cups or molds.

**5.** Place the filled muffin pan or molds in the freezer for 45 minutes or in the refrigerator for 2 hours to firm up.

**6.** Store uneaten fudge in the refrigerator.

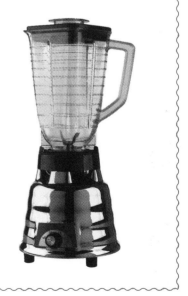

## COCONUT PECAN CHOCOLATE TRUFFLES

*MAKES 8 TRUFFLES*

This tasty truffle recipe relies heavily on coconut and provides a hefty dose of fiber and protein, thanks to the nuts and seeds. I like to wear food gloves when I prepare these treats, since truffle-making is a messy business!

- *1  cup raw pepitas*
- *1  cup raw pecans or walnuts*
- *3  tablespoons coconut nectar*
- *1  teaspoon vanilla extract*
- *1  teaspoon cinnamon*
- *¼  teaspoon salt*
- *2  tablespoons coconut oil*
- *¼  cup unsweetened shredded dried coconut (preferably finely shredded)*

**1.** Line a baking sheet with wax paper. Set aside.

**2.** In the bowl of a food processor, pulse together the pepitas and pecans until they are coarsely chopped.

**3.** Add coconut nectar, vanilla extract, cinnamon, salt, and coconut oil, pulsing until they form a rough paste.

**4.** Using a tablespoon or a small cookie scoop, take a clump of the truffle paste and roll it into a smooth ball. Repeat until all the paste has been used. Place truffle balls on prepared baking sheet.

**5.** Place baking sheet in the refrigerator for 1 hour or until truffle balls are firm.

**6.** Place dried coconut in a shallow bowl or plate. Remove baking sheet from the refrigerator. Roll each truffle ball, one at a time, in the coconut until thoroughly coated. Place truffles back on prepared baking sheet.

**7.** Return to the refrigerator for another hour so they can re-firm after being rolled in coating.

## PUMPKIN COCONUT FUDGE

*MAKES 12 PIECES*

Pumpkin provides beta-carotene for a healthy immune system, eyes, and skin, and coconut offers medium chain fatty acids for cardiovascular health and lauric acid for nervous system function. If you happen to have a blend of pumpkin pie spice in your cupboard, you can use 1 to 2 teaspoons of it instead of the spices listed here, and make Pumpkin Coconut Fudge a new Thanksgiving tradition.

- *¾  cup pumpkin puree (or canned puree)*
- *¾  cup coconut butter*
- *3  tablespoons maple syrup or raw honey*
- *1  teaspoon ground cinnamon*
- *¼  teaspoon ground nutmeg*
- *¼  teaspoon ground ginger*
- *¼  teaspoon ground cloves*

1. Prepare a mini-muffin pan by lining it with muffin papers.

2. In a saucepan over medium heat, mix together all ingredients, stirring until thoroughly combined.

3. Pour mixture into prepared mini-muffin cups.

4. Place the pan in the refrigerator for 1 or more hours to firm up.

5. Store uneaten fudge in a covered container in the refrigerator.

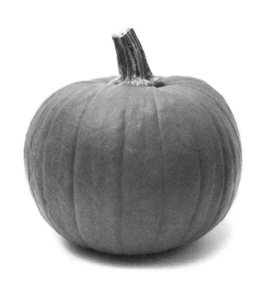

## NUT BUTTER FUDGE

*MAKES 8 PIECES*

Here is yet another coconut fudge recipe that is easy, filling, delicious, and good for you, thanks to all of the healthy coconut (great for cardiovascular, immune, and nervous systems) plus protein-packed nut butter. This recipe comes together very quickly!

½ cup unsalted smooth almond or cashew butter

½ cup coconut butter

¼ cup coconut sugar

¼ cup coconut nectar, Grade B maple syrup, or honey

1 teaspoon vanilla extract

¼ teaspoon salt

1. Lightly grease a mini (5½-by-3-by-2½-inch) loaf pan with coconut oil.

2. In a small pot set over low heat, stir together all ingredients, stirring continually until smooth and completely blended.

3. Pour mixture into prepared pan, smoothing the top with a spatula.

4. Refrigerate 2 hours or until completely firm.

5. Cut into slices to serve.

6. Store uneaten fudge in the refrigerator.

## COOKIES

### COCO-CHIP GLUTEN-FREE COOKIES

*MAKES 12 COOKIES*

Are you gluten-free? You are going to love this chocolate chip cookie recipe. It is delicious and, yep, the coconut flour and coconut oil make it health-supportive, too!

8   *tablespoons semisolid coconut oil*

1   *cup coconut sugar*

1   *egg*

1½ *teaspoons vanilla extract*

½   *cup coconut flour*

½   *cup gluten-free all-purpose flour (can be substituted with regular all-purpose flour if cookies don't need to be gluten-free)*

½   *teaspoon baking soda*

    *Pinch of salt*

1   *cup dark chocolate chips*

**1.** Preheat oven to 375°F.

**2.** Line a baking sheet with foil or parchment.

**3.** In the bowl of a stand mixer, using a paddle attachment, beat together semisolid coconut oil and coconut sugar until well mixed.

**4.** Beat in egg and vanilla.

**5.** In a separate bowl, whisk together coconut flour, gluten-free all-purpose flour, baking soda, and salt.

**6.** Add flour mixture to the ingredients in the bowl of the mixer, and beat on low. Continue until dough is just combined.

**7.** Add chocolate chips and mix just until distributed.

**8.** Using a small ice cream scoop or a teaspoon, drop the dough onto a cookie sheet, about 2 inches apart.

**9.** Bake for 9 to 11 minutes on center rack until just golden.

**10.** Allow cookies to cool on the cookie sheet before removing.

---

#### HOW TO MAKE SEMISOLID COCONUT OIL

To make the semisolid coconut oil called for in several of this book's recipes, simply place your jar or tub of coconut oil in the refrigerator for 30 to 60 minutes. When you remove the coconut oil from the fridge, you'll find it in a soft semisolid state. To measure, spoon what you need into a measuring cup and add to your recipe.

## COCONUT SUGAR COOKIES

*MAKES 5 DOZEN 4-INCH COOKIES*

This coconut-rich cookie is a delicious take on the standard sugar cookie. Try it the next time you want to bake holiday cookies. I like to mix things up by grating in some lemon zest.

- *1 cup semisolid coconut oil*
- *1 cup coconut sugar*
- *1 egg*
- *1 tablespoon canned coconut milk (or regular dairy whole milk)*
- *1 teaspoon vanilla*
- *3 cups all-purpose flour*
- *¾ teaspoon baking powder*
- *½ teaspoon salt*

**1.** In the bowl of a stand mixer, using a paddle attachment, cream together semisolid coconut oil and sugar until light and fluffy.

**2.** Blend in egg, milk, and vanilla until combined.

**3.** In a separate bowl, whisk together flour, baking powder, and salt.

**4.** Slowly, 1 cup at a time, add dry ingredients to the mixing bowl. Mix until just combined.

**5.** Place 2 large sheets of plastic wrap (each about 20 inches long) on a flat, damp surface. Divide dough between sheets of plastic. Pat each into a flat oval, about ½-inch thick.

Cover with more plastic wrap and place in the freezer until firm, about 30 minutes.

**6.** When ready to bake, preheat oven to 375°F.

**7.** Prepare baking sheet with foil or parchment.

**8.** Remove dough from refrigerator or freezer and, using a rolling pin, roll dough about ⅛-inch thick.

**9.** Cut into shapes with cookie cutters.

**10.** Place cookies onto prepared baking sheet about 1 inch apart.

**11.** Bake 8 to 10 minutes or until cookies become golden around the edges.

**12.** Allow cookies to cool thoroughly before decorating them with your favorite toppings—or enjoy them just as they are.

## NUT BUTTER COOKIES

*MAKES 12 COOKIES*

This is my family's go-to cookie. It's gluten-free, super high in protein and fiber, outrageously simple to make, and very tasty. Oh, and it's flexible, too. Sometimes we add some chopped chocolate to the batter or insert a piece of chocolate into thumbprints in the dough. Sometimes I roll these versatile cookies in sugar, cinnamon sugar, finely shredded coconut, or chopped nuts. I tend to make batches of the dough ahead of time and keep it in airtight containers in the fridge for fast treats.

1 cup thick nut butter (peanut, almond, cashew, sunflower, etc.; you can also use a blend of nut butters)

1 cup coconut sugar (you can also use regular sugar or brown sugar or a blend)

1 large egg

½ teaspoon baking soda

Optional: pinch of cinnamon, allspice, or pumpkin pie spice blend

**1.** Preheat oven to 350°F.

**2.** Line a baking sheet with foil or parchment.

**3.** In the bowl of a stand mixer, using the paddle attachment, cream together nut butter and sugar on medium speed until light and fluffy.

**4.** Add in egg, baking soda, and spice, if using. Blend on low speed until just combined.

**5.** Cover dough and chill in the refrigerator until firm, about 30 minutes.

**6.** Form dough into cookies using a cookie scoop or 2 tablespoons. For a fancier look, you can shape into a ball, then press with the tines of a fork to create a classic peanut butter cookie appearance.

**7.** Bake for 8 to 10 minutes or until edges are golden.

**8.** Allow cookies to cool before removing them from baking sheet.

# CARROT OATMEAL COOKIES

*MAKES 18 COOKIES*

I adore sneaking shredded carrots into baked goods. I literally use the pulp leftover when I juice carrots—it works beautifully. In addition to carrots, this wholesome recipe contains oats, walnuts, and coconut oil, creating a cookie filled with fiber, omega-3 fatty acids, medium chain fatty acids, and a bevy of antioxidants. It makes a great addition to any lunch box. Note that this recipe is vegan, making it perfect for those who are allergic to eggs and dairy.

1 cup whole wheat pastry flour or all-purpose flour

1 cup rolled oats

1 teaspoon baking powder

Optional: 1 teaspoon ground cinnamon or pumpkin pie spice blend

¼ teaspoon salt

⅔ cup chopped walnuts (feel free to experiment with other nuts)

1 cup finely shredded carrots

½ cup Grade B maple syrup

½ cup liquid coconut oil

**1.** Preheat oven to 350°F.

**2.** Line a baking sheet with foil or parchment paper.

**3.** In a large bowl, whisk together flour, oats, baking powder, cinnamon (if desired), and salt.

**4.** Stir in nuts and carrots. Set aside.

**5.** In the bowl of a stand mixer, blend together maple syrup and coconut oil until thoroughly combined.

**6.** Add the flour mixture to the syrup-oil mixture, blending on low, until just thoroughly combined.

**7.** Using a cookie scoop or 2 tablespoons, drop dough onto prepared baking sheets, leaving 1½ inches or more of space between them (this cookie spreads).

**8.** Bake until cookies are golden, about 12 to 15 minutes.

**9.** Allow cookies to cool on baking sheet before removing.

## PEANUT-OAT-QUINOA COOKIES

*MAKES 12 COOKIES*

Here is yet another high-protein, high-fiber, nutty, yummy, not-too-sweet coconut-rich cookie! What makes this one a bit different is the quinoa flakes.

**NOTE:** To make these gluten-free, be sure to buy gluten-free oats and gluten-free oat bran. Gluten-free oat products are processed in dedicated, no-gluten facilities.

- ½ *cup oat bran*
- ¼ *cup old-fashioned rolled oats*
- ¼ *cup quinoa flakes*
- ¼ *cup coconut sugar*
- ½ *teaspoon baking powder*
- ¼ *teaspoon salt*
- ½ *teaspoon cinnamon, allspice, or pumpkin pie spice blend*
- ¼ *cup thick peanut butter*
- 1 *large egg*
- ¼ *cup applesauce, pear sauce, or pureed banana*
- 2 *tablespoons Grade B maple syrup*

**1.** Preheat oven to 350°F.

**2.** Line a baking sheet with parchment paper and set aside.

**3.** In a large mixing bowl, whisk together oat bran, rolled oats, quinoa flakes, coconut sugar, baking powder, salt, and spice. Set aside.

**4.** In the bowl of a stand mixer, blend together on a low speed peanut butter, egg, applesauce, and maple syrup.

**5.** Add the dry ingredients to the wet ingredients and blend until thoroughly combined.

**6.** Using a cookie scoop or 2 tablespoons, scoop dough onto prepared cookie sheet. If desired, flatten cookies with the back of a fork.

**7.** Bake until golden, 13 to 15 minutes.

**8.** Allow cookies to cool before removing from baking sheet.

## NO-BAKE COCONUT MACAROONS

*MAKES 12 MACAROONS*

This no-bake recipe is perfect for those times you want something sweet that also has a bit of substance. You'll feel pleasantly full and get a nice steady drip of energy from these macaroons, thanks to the almonds and protein-packed chia. Sometimes I replace the vanilla with ¼ teaspoon of almond extract. Give it a try.

- 1   *tablespoon ground chia seeds*
- 3   *tablespoons warm water*
- 1½ *cups unsweetened shredded dried coconut*
- ½   *cup almonds*
- 10 *Medjool dates, pitted*
- 1   *tablespoon liquid coconut oil*
- 1   *teaspoon vanilla extract*

**1.** In a bowl, whisk together ground chia and warm water. Set aside.

**2.** In a food processor, pulse the coconut and almonds into a fine powder.

**3.** Add the dates, chia mixture, coconut oil, and vanilla. Pulse just until the mixture starts to come together.

**4.** Using a tablespoon, form the mixture into balls and place them on a baking sheet or plate.

**5.** Refrigerate for 30 minutes or more until the macaroons are firm.

## VEGAN OATMEAL COOKIES

*MAKES 18 COOKIES*

This yummy oatmeal-coconut cookie is vegan—perfect for those of you who don't use dairy milk or eat eggs. Applesauce adds extra nutrients and gives the cookies a lovely moist texture.

- 1   *cup whole wheat pastry flour or spelt flour*
- 1   *cup old-fashioned rolled oats*
- 1½ *cups raisins (or chopped dried fruit of choice)*
- 1   *cup unsweetened shredded dried coconut*
- ½   *teaspoon baking soda*
- 1   *teaspoon ground cinnamon*
- 1   *teaspoon ground cardamom (or pumpkin pie spice or allspice)*
  *Pinch of salt*
- ½   *cup applesauce*
- ½   *cup coconut sugar*
- ⅓   *cup coconut nectar or Grade B maple syrup*
- 1   *teaspoon vanilla extract*

**1.** Preheat oven to 350°F.

**2.** Line a baking sheet with foil or parchment.

**3.** In a large bowl, whisk together flour, oats, raisins, shredded coconut, baking soda, cinnamon, cardamom, and salt.

**4.** In a separate bowl, stir together applesauce, coconut sugar, coconut nectar, and vanilla.

**5.** Slowly add the dry ingredients to the wet, stirring until ingredients are thoroughly combined.

**6.** Make cookies using a cookie scoop or 2 tablespoons, placing each on prepared cookie sheet.

**7.** Bake for 15 minutes or until cookies are golden.

**8.** Allow cookies to cool before removing them from baking sheet.

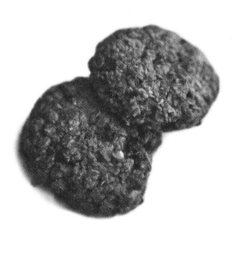

## FROZEN DELIGHTS

### CHOCOLATE-COCONUT BANANAS

*MAKES 12 PIECES*

Two of my sons love bananas. They love them even more if they are accompanied by chocolate (and coconut), hence this homemade version of chocolate-covered bananas.

**NOTE:** You'll need 12 ice-pop sticks or bamboo skewers to make these treats.

- ¼ *cup unsweetened shredded dried coconut*
- 4 *large ripe bananas, peeled, and cut into thirds crosswise*
- ¾ *cup semisweet or bittersweet chocolate chips, melted in a double boiler, slightly cooled*

**1.** Line a baking sheet with parchment, foil, or wax paper. Set aside.

**2.** Spread shredded coconut onto a plate or in a shallow dish. Set aside.

**3.** Insert an ice-pop stick into each piece of banana.

**4.** Working with one piece of banana at a time, dip (or coat, if that's easier) fruit in melted chocolate; then press into shredded coconut.

**5.** Place fully coated banana pieces onto prepared baking sheets and freeze overnight or until frozen.

## SUPERFOOD FREEZER FUDGE

*MAKES 12 PIECES*

Eat this fudge and you get protein, fiber, fatty acids, antioxidants, and loads of phytonutrients. Feel free to play with the nut butter. For a fancier finish, sprinkle coarsely or finely chopped nuts, shredded coconut, or chopped chocolate over the top of the fudge before placing it in the freezer.

- 1   cup almond butter
- 4   tablespoons liquid coconut oil
- 1½ tablespoons coconut nectar or Grade B maple syrup
- 4   ounces 70 percent cacao dark chocolate, melted in a double boiler
- ¼   teaspoon salt

**1.** Lightly grease an 8-by-8-inch baking pan with coconut oil or line it with foil.

**2.** In the bowl of a stand mixer, cream almond butter, coconut oil, coconut nectar, melted chocolate, and salt.

**3.** Pour the mixture into the prepared pan.

**4.** Place the pan in the freezer overnight.

**5.** Remove the pan from freezer, and carefully cut fudge into 12 squares.

**6.** Store uneaten fudge in the freezer.

## FRUITY COCONUT POPS

*MAKES 12 POPS*

My kids—like most kids, I suppose—love frozen treats. Ice pops are a favorite. This recipe is as flexible as you'd like it to be: Use whatever fresh or frozen fruit you have on hand. Coconut milk gives the treats protein and a host of nutrients for stronger immune systems, better brain function, and healthy hearts.

**NOTE:** You'll need 12 ice-pop molds and sticks to make these.

- 1   14-ounce can coconut milk (do not use "lite")
- 1   tablespoon coconut oil
- ¼   cup coconut sugar or cane sugar
- 1   cup chopped fruit of choice

**1.** In a high-speed blender or a food processor, process coconut milk, coconut oil, and sugar until smooth.

**2.** Add fruit and blend until fruit is liquefied—or, if you prefer, almost liquefied. (You may want a few small chunks of fruit in your ice pops.)

**3.** Pour liquid into ice pop molds and insert sticks. Set in the freezer overnight or until frozen solid.

# COCONUT ICE CREAM

*MAKES 6 SERVINGS*

I buy ice cream on only the rarest of occasions. My kids are all semiprofessional singers, and mainstream ice cream means dairy. Which means mucus. Which means struggling through rehearsals and performances. This beautiful confection, however, is always welcome in my freezer. Made with coconut milk, it supports my children's health without any bothersome side effects. You will need an ice cream maker for this one.

2   *14-ounce cans coconut milk*

¾   *cup unsweetened shredded dried coconut*

2   *tablespoons arrowroot starch or cornstarch*

¾   *cup coconut sugar or cane sugar*

 *Pinch of salt*

 *Optional: 1 or more teaspoons vanilla extract*

 *Optional add-ins: ½ to 1 cup chopped nuts, chocolate, fruit, etc.*

**1.** In a blender or food processor, process 1 can of coconut milk with the shredded coconut and arrowroot starch. Set aside.

**2.** In a small saucepan, whisk together the second can of coconut milk, sugar, and salt over medium heat. Bring to a simmer.

**3.** Add the coconut milk mixture from the blender to the saucepan of coconut milk, sugar, and salt. Cook for 2 minutes or until slightly thickened.

**4.** Remove from heat and, if desired, stir in vanilla extract.

**5.** Allow mixture to cool in the refrigerator until thoroughly chilled, about 3 to 4 hours.

**6.** Using an ice cream maker, according to the manufacturer's directions, add chilled coconut mixture and any optional add-ins.

**7.** Freeze the mixture in ice cream maker, according to the manufacturer's instructions.

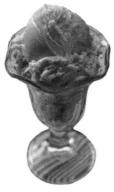

## ARROWROOT POWDER

Arrowroot powder—also known as arrowroot starch—is derived from a tropical South American tuber. Like cornstarch, it is used as a thickener in recipes. The plant was given the name "arrowroot" by the native Caribbean Arawak people, because they used it to draw poison from wounds inflicted by poisoned arrows. Arrowroot was also a foundational food for the Arawak.

## PINEAPPLE-COCONUT SORBET

*MAKES 6 SERVINGS*

I love this healthy, flavorful recipe (it's also rich in antioxidants from the coconut, ginger, and pineapple). An ice cream maker makes the smoothest sorbet, but you can use the "freezer tray method" outlined below.

- ½ cup coconut milk (canned or homemade)
- ½ cup coconut sugar or cane sugar
- 1-inch length of peeled fresh ginger, grated
- 1 whole pineapple (about 3½ pounds), peeled, cored, and cut into chunks
- 1 tablespoon lemon or lime juice

**1.** In a small saucepan over medium heat, whisk together coconut milk, sugar, and ginger. Bring to a simmer for 1 to 2 minutes. Remove from heat and let stand for 20 minutes.

**2.** Place pineapple and lemon juice in a food processor and process until absolutely smooth.

**3.** Add the cooled coconut milk mixture to the pineapple and process until thoroughly blended.

**4.** Pour mixture into ice cream maker and process according to manufacturer's directions. (Alternatively, freeze mixture in a shallow metal pan until solid, about 6 hours. Break into chunks and process in a food processor until smooth. Then pack into an airtight freezer container.)

## COCONUT FUDGE ICE POPS

*MAKES 8 POPS*

The problem with commercial brand fudge pops is the ingredients: high fructose corn syrup, polysorbate 80, polysorbate 65? You don't need to put ingredients like those in your body. Try this healthful version instead. Not only is it tasty; it is good for you!

- 1 14-ounce can coconut milk
- ¼ cup unsweetened cocoa powder
- 3 tablespoons coconut or cane sugar
- 2 teaspoons vanilla extract
- Pinch of salt

**1.** Combine all ingredients in a blender and pulse a few times to blend thoroughly.

**2.** Pour mixture into ice-pop molds and freeze overnight.

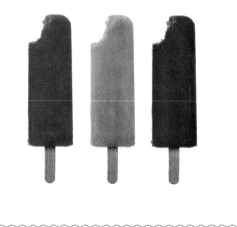

## KEY LIME SUPERFOOD POPS

*MAKES 8 POPS*

Now this is a fun recipe—one truly deserving of the title "superfood," thanks to its blend of avocado and coconut, both of which are known for their extremely beneficial fats, which also nourish the brain, heart, and skin. But, before you ask, no, you cannot taste the avocado. What you can taste, however, is the bright, refreshing flavor of key limes.

**NOTE:** You'll need 8 ice-pop molds and ice-pop sticks when making these treats.

- 1   *avocado, peeled and pitted*
- ½   *cup coconut milk (canned or fresh)*
- ¼   *cup coconut nectar*
- ¼   *cup key lime juice (you can use lemon if you'd like)*
- 2   *teaspoons vanilla extract*
- ¼   *teaspoon salt*

**1.** Process all ingredients in a blender until thoroughly integrated and smooth.

**2.** Pour mixture into ice-pop molds and freeze overnight, or until solid.

## SUMMERTIME MANGO COCONUT SORBET

*MAKES 6 SERVINGS*

Mango is a natural sorbet ingredient—it is both sweet and tart and has a gorgeous bright color that doesn't go away, even when frozen. I like it because it is filled with fiber and vitamin A, for healthy skin and vision. It pairs beautifully with coconut in this elegant recipe. You will love this!

- 2   *cups of chopped mango*
- 1   *14-ounce can coconut milk (do not use "lite")*
- 3   *tablespoons lime juice*
- 3   *tablespoons coconut sugar*
- 1   *tablespoon arrowroot powder*

**1.** In a food processor or high-power blender (such as a Vitamix or Blendtec), puree mango until it becomes a smooth, creamy liquid.

**2.** Add in coconut milk, lime juice, coconut sugar, and arrowroot powder, and pulse just until ingredients are combined.

**3.** Pour liquid into an ice cream maker and freeze according to manufacturer's instructions.

## BERRY MACAROON TART

*MAKES 8 SERVINGS*

Berries and coconut—what a glorious combination! Not only does this taste like summer, but it is also filled with antioxidants and fiber from both the berries and the coconut. You will adore this! It's pretty easy to make, too.

Crust

1 *cup plus 2 tablespoons spelt flour*

½ *cup plus 1 tablespoon dried unsweetened shredded coconut*

½ *cup plus 1 tablespoon regular cane or coconut sugar*

   *Optional: 1 teaspoon lemon or lime zest*

   *Pinch of salt*

6 *tablespoons liquid coconut oil*

Filling

3 *large egg whites*

1½ *cups dried unsweetened shredded coconut*

6 *tablespoons sugar*

6 *to 8 ounces fresh blackberries, raspberries, or other berries, or a mix*

**1.** Preheat oven to 350°F.

**2.** Prepare a 9-inch tart pan by lining the bottom with parchment.

**3.** To make the crust: In a medium bowl, whisk together flour, coconut, sugar, zest, and salt.

**4.** Stir in coconut oil until combined and mixture gets clumpy.

**5.** Press mixture firmly into the bottom of the tart pan, working mixture up the sides of the pan as well. Use the back of a spoon or the bottom of a heavy glass to tamp down crust.

**6.** Place pan on a middle rack in the oven and bake for 15 minutes, or until just golden. Remove pan from oven and allow to cool.

**7.** To make macaroon filling: In a medium bowl, whisk egg whites until light and slightly frothy.

**8.** Stir in coconut and sugar. Set aside.

**9.** Start assembling the tart by scattering the berries over the tart crust.

**10.** Using a teaspoon, drop spoonfuls of the batter over berries. Do not smooth (yes, you want the macaroon batter to remain in lumps).

**11.** Bake for 20 minutes or until macaroon topping begins to turn golden.

**12.** Remove tart from oven and allow to cool before serving.

# CHOCOLATE CREAM TART

*MAKES 8 SERVINGS*

This is basically what my six-year-old calls a "refrigerator pie." But it is so much healthier than the graham cracker crust, boxed pudding mix filling, and whipped topping from a tub that our moms and grandmothers used to make. This one actually has healthy ingredients, including walnuts (omega-3 fatty acids and protein), dates (fiber and minerals), avocado (vitamin K, and folate), and coconut (lauric acid, medium chain fatty acids, and antiviral properties).

- 1 cup walnuts
- 1 cup dates
- 1 ripe avocado
- 2 tablespoons coconut oil
- 2 tablespoons coconut nectar
- 2 tablespoons cocoa powder
- 1 teaspoon vanilla extract
-   Pinch of salt
- ¼ cup canned coconut milk, as needed
-   Optional: 1 cup Coconut Cream Dessert Topping (see page 155)

**1.** Lightly grease a 6-inch or 8-inch tart pan with coconut oil. Set aside.

**2.** To make the crust: In a food processor, pulse the walnuts into powder, then add the dates until it all begins to stick together. Press into prepared tart pan and set aside in the fridge.

**3.** To make the filling: In a clean food processor bowl, add avocado, coconut oil, coconut nectar, cocoa powder, vanilla, and salt. Process until all ingredients are smooth and thick. If filling mixture is too thin, add some coconut milk 1 tablespoon at a time, until you get the right consistency.

**4.** Remove tart pan from the fridge and fill with filling.

**5.** If desired, make the Coconut Cream Dessert Topping (see page 155) and spread 1 cup of it over the tart.

**6.** Place dessert back in the fridge until firm, about an hour.

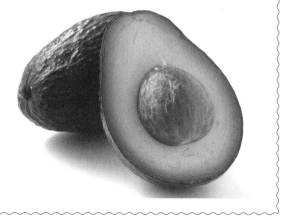

# COCONUT-BASED PIECRUSTS

## NO-BAKE PIECRUST

*MAKES ONE 8-INCH TART CRUST OR PIECRUST*

This yummy, highly nutritious crust is great for unbaked fillings.

2   *cups pitted dates*

2   *cups raw nuts (you can use a blend of nuts)*

¼   *cup unsweetened shredded dried coconut*

½   *teaspoon pumpkin pie spice*

**1.** Prepare an 8-inch tart or pie pan by very lightly greasing with coconut oil. Set aside.

**2.** Add dates to the bowl of a food processor and pulse until coarsely chopped. Remove dates and set aside.

**3.** Wipe out food processor bowl.

**4.** To the clean food processor bowl, add raw nuts, dried coconut, and spice. Pulse a few times, just until it forms a coarse meal.

**5.** Add the dates to the nut-coconut mixture in the food processor. Pulse a few times until a ball forms.

**6.** Spread mixture into the bottom and up the sides of the prepared pie or tart pan, tamping it down to create a uniformly even crust.

**7.** Cover with plastic wrap and refrigerate until ready to be filled.

# COCONUT-BASED PIECRUSTS

Need a coconut-based piecrust? Try one of these!

## ALL-PURPOSE COCONUT-BASED PIECRUST

*MAKES ONE 8-INCH PIECRUST*

Use this buttery-tasting shell for baked or no-bake fillings.

2  *eggs*

1  *cup coconut flour*

½  *cup unsweetened shredded dried coconut*

1  *teaspoon coconut nectar or honey*

   *Pinch of salt*

¼  *cup melted butter*

2  *tablespoons liquid coconut oil*

1  *tablespoon water*

1  *egg white*

**1.** Preheat oven to 350°F.

**2.** In a large bowl, stir together the 2 eggs, coconut flour, shredded coconut, honey, and salt until thoroughly combined.

**3.** Add butter, coconut oil, and water. Mix dough together with a dough cutter or your hands until blended.

**4.** Pat dough into a pie pan, pressing dough firmly into the pan. Use the bottom of a heavy glass to help flatten dough. Set aside.

**5.** Beat egg white with a fork until frothy. Using a pastry brush or your fingers, very lightly brush crust with egg white.

**6.** Place piecrust on a center rack in the oven and bake for 12 to 14 minutes, until barely golden, unless you are using it for a refrigerated pie, in which case bake piecrust until thoroughly golden.

**7.** Cool thoroughly before using.

## PUMPKIN COCONUT PIE

*MAKES 8 SERVINGS*

This is my favorite pumpkin pie—not only do I make it every year for Thanksgiving and Christmas; I make it almost weekly during the fall. It's that easy. My sons love this pie as an afternoon snack. I feel good about serving it, thanks to the high beta-carotene content, as well as the lauric acid from the coconut. If you have pumpkin pie spice blend, use 2½ teaspoons of that instead of the spices given in the ingredient list below.

**NOTE:** The coconut flavor is very light in this. You may not taste it at all.

1   *15-ounce can pumpkin puree*

¾   *cup canned coconut milk (do not use "lite")*

2   *large eggs*

1   *cup packed light brown sugar*

½   *teaspoon salt*

1   *teaspoon grated fresh ginger*

1   *teaspoon cinnamon*

⅛   *teaspoon freshly grated nutmeg*
    *Optional: 1 teaspoon vanilla*
    *Optional: ½ teaspoon lemon zest*

1   *prepared 8-inch or 9-inch pie shell*

**1.** Preheat oven to 400°F.

**2.** In the bowl of a stand mixer, combine pumpkin puree, coconut milk, eggs, brown sugar, salt, spices, and, if desired, vanilla and lemon zest. Mix until smooth and thoroughly combined.

**3.** Pour filling into prepared crust and bake on a middle rack for 45 to 55 minutes or until filling begins to set. (Note: Because this is a custard pie, the center should still be a bit jiggly when you remove the pie; it will firm up as it cools.)

**4.** Allow to cool 2 hours at room temperature or in the refrigerator before serving.

## COCONUT CREAM PIE

*MAKES 8 SERVINGS*

This coconut cream pie is very much like a traditional coconut cream pie, except that it's made with a coconut flour crust (you can use a premade regular pie shell, if you like) and the filling features raw coconut and coconut cream topping. Coconut lovers will go wild for this!

1   *coconut-based piecrust (see recipes in sidebar on pages 150–151), cooled, or 1 premade 8-inch pie shell*

3   *egg yolks*

1½  *cups raw young coconut flesh*

½   *cup raw honey*
    *Pinch of salt*

⅓   *cup coconut water or regular water*

1½  *tablespoons unflavored powdered gelatin*

½   *cup coconut cream*

*Optional garnish: 1 cup Coconut Cream Dessert Topping (see page 155)*

*Optional garnish: ¼ cup toasted coconut for topping (see sidebar)*

**1.** Make piecrust according to one of the recipes on pages 150–151 if you are opting for homemade.

**2.** Preheat oven to 350°F.

**3.** In the bowl of a food processor or blender, add egg yolks, raw coconut meat, raw honey, and salt. Process until mixture is creamy and smooth.

**4.** Heat coconut water in a small saucepan until boiling. Remove from heat and whisk in gelatin. Allow to cool for 3 minutes.

**5.** Add gelatin mixture to the coconut filling in the food processor and blend until gelatin is mixed through.

**6.** Scrape filling into a mixing bowl and set aside.

**7.** In the bowl of a stand mixer, using a whisk attachment, beat coconut cream and whip until soft peaks form.

**8.** Gently fold cream into coconut filling.

**9.** Scrape pie filling into cooled crust. Cover pie and place in refrigerator for at least 3 hours to set.

**10.** If desired, dress with whipped coconut topping and/or toasted coconut.

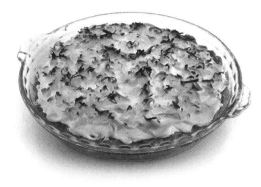

## HOW TO TOAST COCONUT

If you've ever toasted coconut before, you know it can go from light to burnt in an instant. Here are some tips to keep your coconut crunchy, not scorched:

**1.** Preheat your oven to 325°F. Your oven does not need to be a roaring inferno to toast coconut.

**2.** Spread coconut in a single later on a baking sheet.

**3.** Place baking sheet on a middle rack in the oven, and check on it at the 5-minute mark.

**4.** Give the coconut a stir, then check it again in 1 or 2 minutes.

**5.** Continue checking every minute until the coconut is uniformly golden. Don't let it get brown or it will taste bitter.

## APPLE BERRY COCONUT CRISP

*MAKES 4 SERVINGS*

This multi-fruit crumble is flexible: Feel free to substitute pears for the apples, cranberries for the blackberries, and so on.

    5   large cooking apples, chopped
    1   cup water, apple cider, or pear nectar
    2   tablespoons coconut sugar
    1   teaspoon cinnamon
    ½   teaspoon nutmeg
    ¾   cup coconut flour
    ¼   cup unsweetened shredded dried coconut
    3   tablespoons coconut oil
    3   tablespoons Grade B maple syrup
        Dash of salt
    1   cup blackberries

**1.** Preheat oven to 350°F.

**2.** Lightly grease a casserole dish or gratin pan with coconut oil. Set aside.

**3.** Add apples, water, coconut sugar, and spices to a saucepan and simmer over low heat for 5 to 10 minutes, until apples just begin to soften. Remove from heat.

**4.** In a bowl, whisk together the flour, dried coconut, coconut oil, maple syrup, and dash of salt. It should resemble a crumble mixture.

**5.** Add the apple mixture to the prepared pan and gently stir in berries.

**6.** Top fruit with crisp mixture, spreading crumbs evenly across the top.

**7.** Bake for 20 minutes until golden brown and bubbling.

**8.** Remove from oven and allow to cool slightly (about 30 minutes) before serving.

## TWENTY-FIRST-CENTURY AMBROSIA

*MAKES 6 SERVINGS*

If you grew up in the United States, you probably know ambrosia. Mini marshmallows, a can of tangerine sections, and maybe some fruit cocktail topped off with Cool Whip and perhaps some sweetened shredded coconut. My mom would also throw in some pomegranate seeds, since they grew wild on our property. Well, I am here to tell all you healthy eaters out there that ambrosia can have a place in your life—as long as you use a healthy recipe, like this one.

    ½   cup canned coconut milk (do not use "lite")
    ½   tablespoon arrowroot or cornstarch
    3   tablespoons sugar
    ¼   teaspoon pure vanilla extract
        Optional: 1 teaspoon tangerine or orange zest
    1   apple, cored, seeded, and cut into ¼-inch dice
    1   tablespoon lemon juice

½ cup roughly chopped walnuts or pecans

½ cup unsweetened shredded dried coconut

3 tangerines, peel and pith removed, roughly chopped

2 large oranges, peel and pith removed, roughly chopped

**1.** In a large bowl, whisk together coconut milk and arrowroot until smooth.

**2.** Whisk in sugar, vanilla, and if desired, zest until smooth. Set aside.

**3.** In another bowl, gently coat apple pieces with lemon juice to prevent browning.

**4.** To the coconut milk mixture, gently add chopped nuts and dried coconut.

**5.** Fold in apples, tangerines, and oranges until just combined.

**6.** Cover and chill for at least 1 hour before serving.

## COCONUT BANANAS

*MAKES 4 SERVINGS*

This is the perfect after-school snack. It's healthy, sweet, kid-friendly, and easy to make no matter what your age. If you're looking for a fun recipe to make with the kids, try this one.

4 teaspoons cocoa powder

4 teaspoons finely shredded unsweetened dried coconut (pulse shredded coconut in the food processor for a finer texture)

2 small bananas, sliced on the bias

**1.** Place cocoa and coconut on separate plates. Roll each banana slice in the cocoa, shake off the excess, then dip in the coconut. Eat immediately or rest on a plate or sheet of waxed paper and place in the refrigerator until you're ready to enjoy.

### COCONUT CREAM DESSERT TOPPING

Are you looking for a luscious alternative to whipped cream? Look no further! I've got one for you here, and it harnesses the health-supportive benefits of coconut!

To make the topping, take a 14-ounce can of coconut cream (do not use sweetened cream of coconut) and shake it well. Leave the can in the refrigerator overnight, then remove it and shake it well again. Empty the contents into the bowl of a stand mixer, add 1 tablespoon of vanilla extract, and spoon in 1 to 3 tablespoons of powdered sugar. Using the whisk attachment of the mixer, begin to beat the coconut cream and slowly increase the speed to medium. Beat the mixture until the coconut cream looks light and airy, about 3 to 5 minutes. Use this delicious stuff whenever you'd normally use whipped dairy cream.

## SUMMER CRUMBLE

*MAKES 6 SERVINGS*

This is one nutrient-dense crumble! Here are all the good things you'll find inside: hempseed for fiber and protein; oats for fiber; coconut for fiber, antioxidants, and medium chain fatty acids; berries for antioxidants; and almond for protein. This delicious dessert is so healthy you can serve it for breakfast and know your family is getting the nutrients they need. Note that the recipe calls for many of the same ingredients in different measures and places, so follow the instructions carefully.

- 3 cups mixed fresh berries
- 2 tablespoons lemon juice
- 1 tablespoon plus 1 teaspoon vanilla extract
- 9 tablespoons coconut sugar, divided
- 1 teaspoon coconut flour plus ¼ cup
- ¼ cup almond flour
- ¼ cup rolled oats, quick style
- 2 tablespoons unsweetened shredded coconut
- ¼ cup hempseed
- ½ teaspoon cinnamon
- ½ teaspoon ginger
    Pinch of salt
- ½ cup liquid coconut oil

**1.** Preheat oven to 350°F.

**2.** Lightly grease a casserole or gratin dish with coconut oil. Set aside.

**3.** Gently toss the berries in a mixing bowl with the lemon juice, 1 tablespoon of the vanilla, 4 tablespoons of the coconut sugar, and 1 teaspoon of the coconut flour. Let stand.

**4.** To make the crumble: Whisk together the remaining coconut flour, almond flour, oats, shredded coconut, hempseed, remaining 5 tablespoons coconut sugar, cinnamon, ginger, and salt in a bowl.

**5.** In a separate small bowl, whisk together coconut oil and the remaining 1 teaspoon of vanilla. Drizzle this over the crumble mixture, using your hands or a dough cutter to combine until it takes on the appearance of coarse crumbs.

**6.** Place the berry mixture in the prepared baking dish. Sprinkle the crumble mixture on top.

**7.** Bake until the mixture is bubbling and the top is golden, about 20 to 30 minutes.

**8.** Allow to cool to room temperature before serving. Serve as is, or with Coconut Cream Dessert Topping (see page 155).

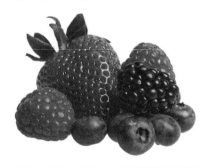

## PUDDINGS

## BROWN RICE COCONUT PUDDING

*MAKES 4 SERVINGS*

I learned this recipe in cooking school, but many people (including food writer Mark Bittman) offer similar versions. Yes, it's that good.

- ⅓ cup uncooked long-grain brown rice
- 2 14-ounce cans coconut milk (do not use "lite")
- ½ cup coconut sugar, brown sugar, or maple sugar
  Pinch of salt

**1.** Preheat oven to 300°F.

**2.** Add uncooked rice to the bowl of a food processor. Pulse 2 or 3 times, just enough to gently break apart the grains. You don't want to make meal or flour out of them!

**3.** Whisk together coconut milk, sugar, and salt in a large casserole dish or Dutch oven.

**4.** Stir in broken rice and place casserole dish in the oven, uncovered. Bake for 40 minutes. After 40 minutes, open oven and stir pudding mixture 3 times.

**5.** Close oven and allow the pudding to continue baking for an additional 45 minutes. Open oven and stir the pudding again, 3 times.

**6.** Close oven and bake for an additional 40 minutes.

**7.** The pudding is done when the grains are swollen and soft. It may not be completely thickened; the pudding will continue to thicken once it is removed from the oven. If the grains are even a bit al dente, leave the pudding in the oven for another 10 minutes and then check it again.

## PUMPKIN COCONUT MOUSSE

*MAKES 4 SERVINGS*

I have studied health-supportive cooking and also have a pastry degree—two very different cooking school experiences to be sure! One of my favorite pastry school desserts was a pumpkin mousse made with whipping cream, nutmeg, and brown sugar. This recipe is my shot at making a delicious, whole food, healthy version of the original. I'd say I nailed it!

- 1 15-ounce can pureed pumpkin (not the pumpkin pie mix), chilled
- ⅓ cup Grade B maple syrup
- 1 teaspoon vanilla extract
- 2 teaspoons cinnamon
- ¼ teaspoon nutmeg
- ¼ teaspoon ginger
- ¼ teaspoon cloves
- ⅓ cup coconut cream, chilled (not cream of coconut)

1. In the bowl of a stand mixer, mix together pumpkin puree, maple syrup, vanilla, and spices. Beat until smooth and thoroughly blended. Remove bowl and set aside.

2. Set a clean bowl under the mixer. Add the coconut cream. Using a whisk attachment, whip coconut cream 3 or more minutes on medium speed until light and fluffy.

3. Using a large spatula, gently fold whipped coconut cream into pumpkin mixture. Chill in the fridge for 30 minutes, or longer, to allow flavors to blend.

4. Ladle into serving dishes.

## COCONUT QUINOA PUDDING

*MAKES 4 SERVINGS*

When my kids talk about quinoa, they talk about this pudding—which is known as "breakfast quinoa" in my home because I serve it to them in the morning.

1   *14-ounce can coconut milk (not "lite")*

¾   *cup uncooked quinoa (red, white, or tricolor), rinsed and drained*

2   *tablespoons coconut nectar or Grade B maple syrup*

1   *teaspoon vanilla extract*

*Optional garnish: Chopped fruit, dried fruit, sunflower seeds, chopped nuts, shredded coconut, etc.*

1. In a small saucepan over medium-high heat, bring coconut milk and quinoa to a boil.

2. Reduce heat to medium-low and stir in coconut nectar and vanilla.

3. Continue to cook, stirring occasionally, for about 30 minutes, until mixture is creamy and has a pudding-like consistency.

4. Serve warm or allow to cool in the refrigerator.

5. Garnish before serving, if desired.

## CHIA PUDDING

*MAKES 2 SERVINGS*

Protein-rich chia provides an easy, steady supply of energy that works as well for the average person trying to get through the day as it does for an endurance athlete. This sweet and delicious chia pudding makes a lovely afternoon snack. It's also a great way to start the day: My kids sometimes have this for breakfast with a green drink.

⅔   *cup chia seeds*

2   *cups canned or fresh coconut milk*

½   *teaspoon pure vanilla extract*

*Optional sweetener: 1 to 3 teaspoons coconut nectar, honey, maple syrup, or other natural sweetener*

*Optional topping: 2 tablespoons currants or chopped dried figs, or dates, or fresh berries, or diced cooked sweet potato*

*Optional topping: 2 tablespoons unsweetened coconut flakes*

**1.** Put chia seeds, coconut milk, vanilla and, if using, optional sweetener in a 1-quart glass jar with a lid. Tighten the lid and shake well to combine thoroughly. Or stir together these ingredients in a bowl.

**2.** Allow the pudding to thicken for 30 minutes or more. (Or, even better, make the pudding in the evening and let it sit, covered, overnight in the fridge.)

**3.** Adjust liquid if necessary. Spoon the pudding into bowls and top with optional fruit and coconut, if desired.

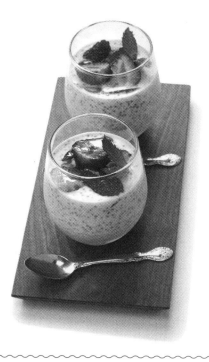

## COCONUT CREAM LIME PUDDING

*MAKES 2 SERVINGS*

Key lime pie is my family's absolute favorite. Looking for a way to get more skin-saving coconut into the diet of my eczema-riddled oldest child, I began playing with coconut-based lime recipes made from whole food ingredients. Here's my attempt. I love it and hope you will, too.

> *Flesh from ½ young coconut*
> 2 *tablespoons liquid coconut oil*
> 1 *to 2 tablespoons coconut nectar*
> 1 *peeled lime*
> *Pinch of salt*
> ½ *teaspoon ginger powder*
> ½ *teaspoon vanilla extract*
> ¼ *cup coconut water, if needed*

**1.** Using a food processor or a high-power blender (such as a Vitamix or Blendtec), blend all the ingredients except coconut water, until smooth and fluffy white.

**2.** Only if the mixture is too thick to blend, add coconut water 1 tablespoon at a time. Blend until incorporated.

**3.** Ladle pudding into dishes and chill for 30 minutes before serving.

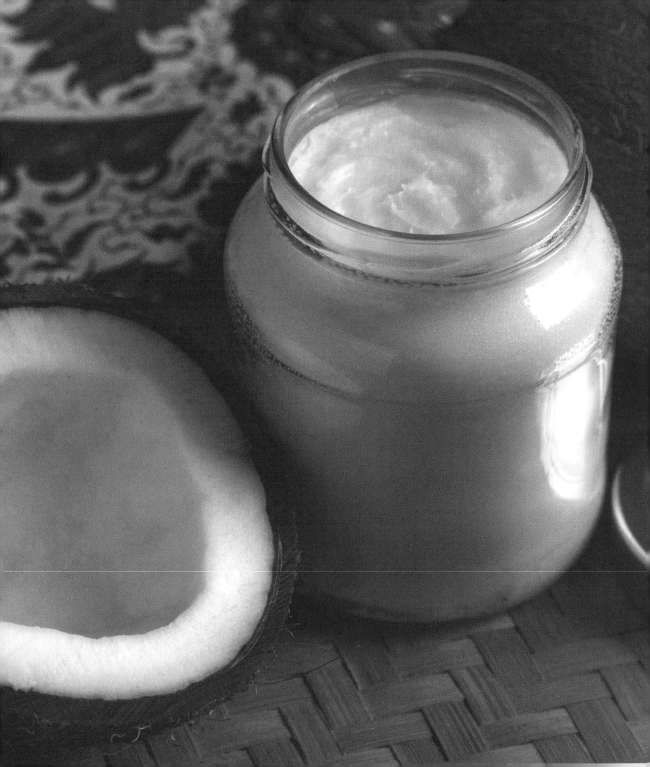

# CHAPTER 9

# FREQUENTLY ASKED QUESTIONS

When an ingredient comes in as many forms as coconut does, there are bound to be questions. Here are some of the coconut questions I am asked most often.

## WHOLE COCONUTS

*How long can I store an unopened green coconut?*

One month or less. That said, whole coconuts do not come with harvest dates or expiration dates, so it's almost impossible to know exactly how old your green coconut is. Furthermore, most coconuts take about one to two months to make it from the plantation in Southeast Asia (where most commercially grown coconuts originate) to a grocery store in North America or Europe. Because most of the coconuts we buy in North America and Europe are grown in Southeast Asia, they may have traveled up to two months before reaching the grocery store. So to be safe, store your green coconut in the fridge to slow down spoilage and use it within five days of buying it.

*Can I tell if a green coconut is spoiled before i open it?*

A green coconut should be heavy with liquid. If you don't hear a sloshing sound when you gently shake it, and if there are any soft or weepy spots on the surface, there's a chance that it is spoiled. If you open the coconut and smell an "off" odor or the liquid is pink, it is spoiled.

*How long can I store an unopened mature coconut?*

About one month or less in a cool place. I'll say the same thing I said about the green, young coconuts: It is impossible to know exactly how old your mature coconut is. Furthermore, most coconuts take about one to two months to make it from the plantation in Southeast Asia (where most commercially grown coconuts originate) to a grocery store in North America or Europe. So to be safe, store your mature coconut in the fridge to slow down spoilage and use it within a week or two of buying it.

*Can I tell if a mature coconut is spoiled before I open it?*

You want a heavy coconut that makes a sloshing sound when you gently shake it. Check the coconut eyes. They should be firm and dry. Any moisture or weepiness in these areas is a bad sign. Check the husk for mold or bald spots or breaks, all of which indicate spoilage.

## COCONUT OIL

*Does coconut oil go rancid easily?*

No, not really. Coconut oil has a long shelf life and can stay fresh for up to three years if it is kept in an airtight container (like a jar) at room temperature or in a cool storage area.

*Some recipes call for semisolid coconut oil. Is this a special type of coconut oil?*

Coconut oil is naturally liquid at temperatures above 75°F. When you see semisolid coconut called for in a recipe, refrigerate it for thirty minutes or more beforehand to allow it to solidify. Then proceed as directed with the recipe.

*Everyone says coconut oil is so great for your skin, but it makes me break out. Is that normal?*

It is normal. It makes me break out, too, in big cystic pimples—on my face. But it does wonders for my feet, legs, hands, arms, and torso! Your face is oilier than other parts of your body and is more prone to clogged pores. It makes sense that applying oil to it could create problems.

*There are so many different types of coconut oil in the store. Which kind should I get?*

I like to go with the purest, least processed product I can find, which in the case of coconut oil, is organic extra-virgin, cold-pressed oil. This means that the coconuts were grown organically and no chemicals and no heat have been used to help extract the oil from the meat.

*My dog loves coconut oil. Is it okay for her to have it?*

Yes. In fact, coconut oil's antimicrobial and antiparasitic qualities make it a great way to help your pooch or even your cat stay healthy. Research has shown that coconut oil kills giardia and other harmful protozoa. The oil also helps digestion and promotes a beautiful coat. For a dog, try 1 teaspoon of oil for every 10 pounds of the dog's weight, once a day, drizzled over food. For cats, try 1 teaspoon of oil a day over food or (if your cat is picky) rubbed into a spot on his or her fur where it will be licked off.

## FRESH COCONUT FLESH

*What's the difference between the interior of a young, green coconut and a mature, brown coconut?*

The flesh from young green coconuts has a slightly translucent, gelatinous texture. As coconuts age, they become starchy. Thus, the interior of mature coconut is more like the meat of a nut: denser, opaque in color, and starchier in taste. Referred to as "coconut meat," it is easily grated or dried.

*Can I dry the flesh from a young, green coconut?*

Because of its soft, jelly-like texture, the flesh from a green coconut doesn't dry well. It is delicious, however, eaten as is or pureed with some fruit and a bit of sweetener as a pudding or added to a smoothie.

*How long can I keep fresh coconut flesh (from a young, green coconut) in the refrigerator?*

Try to use it within two or three days. If you can't, freeze it in an airtight container.

*Is it possible to be allergic to coconut meat?*

Anything is possible! Allergies to coconut meat are rare, but should you experience one, symptoms could be itching, hives, nausea, vomiting, diarrhea, trouble breathing, and swelling of the lips and tongue. Much more common are contact allergies to the outside of the coconut—a form of latex allergy, because the outside of the coconut contains natural latex, and can cause an itchy rash or blisters that develop within a day or two of touching the coconut.

# COCONUT WATER

*Are the packaged coconut waters I see in the store actually raw?*

No, most store-bought packaged coconut waters are not raw. Coconut water is a highly perishable product and to keep it safe and salable, most companies pasteurize it before packaging. As of this book's writing, the only truly raw coconut water I know of is Harmless Harvest Organic 100% Raw Coconut Water, which you can find in the refrigerator case of most mainstream grocers and health food stores.

*I've heard that coconut water spoils easy. I find coconut water to taste weird anyway— how would I even know if it is spoiled?*

You'll know when it's spoiled—it has a sour "off" taste and smell compared to the regular coconut water weird smell. You will definitely know if it's bad!

Here's how to avoid buying spoiled coconut water: When buying boxed or bottled coconut water, always check the expiration date. If the date is close to expiration, don't buy the water. Once you've opened the container, use it within two days.

*Do you have some ideas for using leftover coconut water? My husband always opens up a box, drinks a bit and stashes it in the fridge, never to return to it. I feel bad throwing it away.*

You can use leftover coconut water (as long as it's still fresh!) for part of the liquid in cooking or baking, or you can add it to a smoothie. In my opinion, though, the easiest and most reliable way to use leftover coconut water is to freeze it in an ice cube tray and make coconut water ice cubes. You can use these in smoothies or as a refreshing addition to water, coconut water, or other cool drinks.

*Is it true coconut water can be used in place of plasma if someone needs a transfusion?*

No. There has been one documented case of a man in the Solomon Islands during World War II who received an emergency IV drip of coconut water when regular IV saline solution was unavailable.

## COCONUT FLOUR

*Is coconut flour simply ground-up dried coconut?*

Coconut flour is actually a by-product of coconut milk: To make coconut milk, fresh or dried coconut meat is blended with water. The liquid is then strained and any of the remaining solids—aka "pulp"—is laid out to dry, then ground into flour.

*Why is coconut flour tricky to bake with?*

Coconut flour is extraordinarily high in fiber, so it requires large amounts of liquid ingredients for baked goods. Also, because it's so heavy, coconut flour usually does better when it comprises no more than 20 percent of a recipe.

*What's the best way to store coconut flour?*

Coconut flour can keep for up to a year, if stored in an airtight container in a cool place. I keep mine in the freezer.

## DRIED COCONUT

*Why is dried coconut called "desiccated" coconut?*

The word "desiccated" means "dried."

*Does dried coconut have a shelf life?*

Six months to a year depending upon how warm your kitchen is. For longer storage, keep it in the freezer.

*Why is sweetened flake coconut—which is basically dried coconut with sugar—so much moister than unsweetened dried coconut?*

Sweetened flake coconut is coated in sugar as it dries. Sugar is a humectant, which means that it draws moisture toward it. This is why sweetened flake coconut is typically moist.

# COCONUT MILK

*Is coconut milk the liquid in a mature coconut?*

No. Mature coconuts typically don't contain a lot of liquid—some contain none at all—and what they do contain is not very tasty. Coconut milk is actually a manufactured food, created by mixing together 1½ cups of fresh or dried coconut and about 4 cups of warm water until a creamy white liquid is created. The liquid is then strained to remove any solids—which can be used in baking. Try it yourself if you have time! Just make sure to refrigerate the milk and use it within three days; it spoils quickly.

*What is the difference between coconut milk in cans, boxes, and cartons? And can they be used interchangeably?*

Coconut milk comes packaged in a few different ways: The most common is in cans. But you can also get it in cartons or boxes. While these are all coconut milk, there are some differences, which is why in the recipes throughout this book, you'll often see that I specify what kind of coconut milk works best.

Cans are probably what you know best. Straight coconut milk is packaged in cans—either as is or mixed with a few additives. (These are typically 13.5 to 15 ounces in volume.) Most of the recipes in this book call for regular canned coconut milk. Note: A lot of people ask me about "lite" coconut milk, which has some of the fat removed. I rarely use this and don't call for it in any of this book's recipes. But, if lite coconut milk is all you can find, it will work. Your recipe may not turn out in taste or texture like it would have had you used regular, full-fat coconut milk, but I realize that sometimes you must work with what you have.

A few years back, aseptic boxes of shelf-stable coconut milk beverage began appearing on shelves. Meant to be a dairy-free substitute for cow's milk, these typically contain coconut milk, water, a sweetener of some type, stabilizers, many thickeners, and even flavorings, such as vanilla. And just recently, cartons of these same drinks began appearing in the refrigerator case (near the cow's milk). It's exactly the same product, without the shelf-stable box. I tend not to buy these cartons because they have so many additives, but they work just fine in most recipes for drinks and in recipes that do not require cooking. You'll see a few recipes in this book that mention them as an ingredient alternative.

*What are all the extra ingredients in my can of coconut milk?*

Some brands are 100 percent coconut milk, but many contain thickeners, stabilizers, emulsifiers, and preservatives. Guar gum is the most common preservative; it is used to keep the milk from doing what it wants to do naturally (i.e., separate into a creamy solid at the top and into a milk at the bottom). Guar is a bean that is dehusked and pulverized to create an off-white powder—although seaweed (carrageenan) is sometimes used for this purpose. Other common additives include citric acid (a preservative derived from citrus) and potassium metabisulfite (a laboratory-made preservative).

### What about BPA in the cans used for canned coconut milk?

Some brands of coconut milk use BPA-coated cans, and some don't. I hesitate to offer up brand names because, as I worked on this cookbook, a brand I had long relied on switched to BPA cans, so I am going to ask you, dear reader, to do some research before you buy.

So what is BPA? These letters stand for "bisphenol A," a carbon-based synthetic compound that has been used in industry since the late 1950s to line cans, including cans that contain food. Here's the problem: BPA has been linked with several health conditions, including neuro-behavioral problems, cancer, and infertility.

In tests conducted by the Centers for Disease Control and Prevention (CDC), BPA was found in the urine of 93 percent of adults tested. Fortunately, a study published in Environmental Health Perspectives found that families who ate fresh food (none of it canned), and who used only glass storage containers, experienced a 60 percent reduction of BPA in their urine.

### I've heard there is such a thing as frozen coconut milk, but I've never seen it. Do you know anything about this?

Frozen coconut milk—just coconut milk—that has been flash pasteurized and frozen in plastic packages can be found in some Southeast Asian markets. It isn't widely available and I have yet to see frozen coconut milk in mainstream grocery stores. If you thaw the milk and stir it, it can be used in any of the recipes in this book.

### I was in an Indian grocery store and saw something called powdered coconut milk. What is that?

Before I had children, my husband and I used to spend months at a time in Jamaica for the music, the food, and the island itself. One thing we used to always bring back with us was bags of powdered coconut milk, which we'd buy from the woman who ran the small grocery store down the road from our rental. When friends went back home to Barbados or Trinidad, or traveled in the West Indies, we always asked them to bring dried coconut milk back. I found it—and still find it—outrageously convenient. It is literally dehydrated coconut milk that you stir with water to make as thick or thin as you want. While you probably won't find powdered coconut milk in a mainstream grocery store, search out a store that specializes in Southeast Asian or West

Indian or Indian-Pakistani foods. You'll find it with no problem. Or, order it online. Of course you can always plan to travel to the Caribbean and get it there!

## COCONUT YOGURT

*I've seen coconut yogurt on the market. What is this stuff?*

It is a nondairy yogurt that is made from coconut. In other words, it's a creamy, fermented coconut milk product, and it can be used interchangeably with dairy yogurt in uncooked and cooked recipes. Like dairy yogurt, it comes in unsweetened and sweet flavored versions. Some brands, not wanting to confuse consumers with the word "yogurt," call it "cultured coconut milk."

## COCONUT KEFIR

*I've heard that kefir can be made with coconut. Is it just as healthy as the dairy variety?*

Yes, kefir can be made with either coconut water or coconut milk. And yes, it's just as rich in probiotics as the dairy variety. Coconut water kefir is made from coconut water taken from fresh, green coconuts. This water is fermented, bottled in dark bottles, and kept refrigerated at all times. It is a highly perishable product and is available in the refrigerator cases of most health food stores and some mainstream grocery stores. Coconut milk kefir is more like drinkable yogurt—it is the nondairy version of dairy kefir and comes in unflavored versions and sweetened, flavored varieties. It is not as perishable as coconut water kefir, and it is also high in probiotics. It's great to use in smoothies and uncooked recipes. It is available in most mainstream supermarkets right where you'd expect it: the dairy case.

## COCONUT MILK ICE CREAM

*I have noticed so many coconut "ice creams" on the market. I don't love the taste of coconut but can't have dairy. Have you tried these? Can you tell me if they are overwhelmingly "coconutty" in taste?*

Two of my children don't do well with dairy, which means that, yes, I have tried these coconut milk ice creams. Wow, are they good. So, so much better than the rice milk and almond milk frozen treats! But that doesn't answer your question, does it? You definitely can taste the coconut in the vanilla flavor of every brand I've tried. It's not overwhelming, but it is there. Strawberry, chocolate, mint, and other flavors tend to be free of any coconut taste. I bet you'll love them. Having said that, these are still treat foods, with plenty of sugar, so enjoy in moderation!

## COCONUT NONDAIRY CREAMER

*What is coconut nondairy creamer? I read about it on a blog and am curious.*

I know you've seen this in pint cartons in the dairy case of your local supermarket. Coconut nondairy creamer is basically coconut cream and water with thickeners, stabilizers, and (for some varieties) sweeteners and flavorings. Personally, I avoid this kind of product. If I can't have dairy milk in my tea, then I use straight coconut milk or coconut cream.

## COCONUT NECTAR

*Is coconut nectar sap from the coconut tree?*

Unlike maple syrup, coconut syrup—better known as "nectar"—does not come from bark. It is a liquid that is secreted by the stem of the coconut palm's blossoms.

*Can I bake with coconut nectar?*

Absolutely. Look for recipes developed with coconut nectar in mind, or find recipes that currently use another liquid sweetener and swap in coconut nectar. It can be used in a 1:1 ratio for honey, maple syrup, brown rice syrup, barley malt, and even agave.

*Does coconut nectar have any health benefits?*

Coconut nectar is a rich source of minerals, seventeen amino acids, vitamin C, and B-complex vitamins.

## COCONUT SUGAR

*What is coconut sugar?*

Coconut sugar is coconut nectar that has been dehydrated—just like sugar is cane syrup that has been dehydrated.

*Is coconut sugar the same as palm sugar?*

Sometimes. . . . This can be a bit confusing, so let's see if I can break this down: In Thailand and other Southeast Asian countries, the two words are used to describe coconut sugar. So from brands sourced from those areas, you may see coconut sugar marketed as palm sugar or coconut palm sugar or coconut sugar. It's also known as coco sap sugar or coco sugar. In addition, there is another product, which comes from the sugar palm. It is called palm sugar, too. If you don't like being confused, look specifically for the word "coconut."

*Can I use coconut sugar as a replacement for cane sugar?*

Yes, it can be used, in a 1:1 ratio, as a replacement, but its texture is coarser than that of regular sugar. Just give it a quick pulse in a food processor or coffee grinder to make it finer and easier to incorporate with other ingredients.

*Does coconut sugar have any nutritional benefits?*

Coconut sugar has a high mineral content—so it's a rich source of potassium, magnesium, zinc, and iron. In addition, it contains vitamins B1, B2, B3, and B6. When compared to brown cane sugar, coconut sugar has eighteen times the potassium, thirty times the phosphorus, and over ten times the amount of zinc.

# COCONUT AMINOS

*I don't quite understand this aminos thing. Is coconut aminos like Bragg Liquid Aminos that my vegan friends use?*

Think of coconut aminos as soy sauce without the soy. Soy is an allergen, and there are plenty of people who feel better without it. Coconut aminos, made from the fermented sap of coconut trees and sea salt, offers that same rich, salty, satisfying flavor, but in a more health-supportive way.

How does it compare with Bragg Liquid Aminos? The Bragg product has the same ingredients as soy sauce, but isn't fermented and contains sixteen amino acids that are not present in soy sauce. So if you have issues with soy, you'll have them with Bragg Liquid Aminos, too.

# COCONUT VINEGAR

*I have just bought a bottle of coconut vinegar. It looks like apple cider vinegar—can I use it the same way?*

You're right, the two vinegars do look alike—they are even the same color. Coconut vinegar, made from fermented coconut water, can be used in the same way as apple cider vinegar. I tend to use it (and coconut oil) when I make salad dressings. For those of you who like to mix a splash of apple cider vinegar in water for a refreshing, alkalizing drink, you can also do that with coconut vinegar. You can even cook with coconut vinegar.

# COCONUT BUTTER

*What is coconut butter?*

It is a mixture of coconut oil and dried coconut that has been pureed into a thick, opaque paste, or butter. To try your hand at homemade coconut butter, add equal amounts coconut oil and unsweetened dried coconut to a food processor and process for ten minutes. It should be thick, so add more dried coconut if necessary. Pack the butter into a glass jar or airtight container, and store it in a cool place.

*Is coconut butter the same thing as the coconut manna I have seen produced by one brand?*

Yes. Some brands also call it Coconut Bliss or Coconut Concentrate.

*Are solid coconut oil and coconut butter the same thing?*

No. Solid coconut oil is the oil that is cool enough to solidify (just like "regular" butter, it is solid at certain temperatures and melts in warmer temperatures). Coconut butter is a combination of dried coconut meat and coconut oil, blended together to form a thick, opaque creamy paste. Think peanut or almond oil versus peanut or almond butter. And just so you know, the two are not interchangeable in recipes.

## COCONUT CREAM

*Is coconut cream like whipped cream?*

Not really, though it is like whipping cream! Just like whipping (or heavy) cream, coconut cream is the full-fat (coconut), low-water product—one that actually can be whipped into a vegan whipped cream for desserts. Check out the dessert chapter for a recipe. Coconut cream comes unsweetened in small cans, jars, and squeeze bottles. You can also find it floating as a solid layer on the top of brands of canned coconut milk that do not contain guar gum or other emulsifiers. Do not substitute cream of coconut.

## CREAM OF COCONUT

*I get so confused about canned coconut products. Can you tell me again what cream of coconut is?*

Cream of coconut is a canned, sweetened product, typically found in the same aisle as premade drink mixes and drink syrups. Most brands use a photo of a piña colada or other frozen drink on the label. It is the thick cream you find on the top of unshaken coconut milk mixed with corn syrup or sugar. It is a popular ingredient in sweet coconut-tasting, "tropical" mixed drinks. As I heard one culinary instructor put it: Cream of coconut is to coconut milk what condensed milk is to regular milk. Cream of coconut is a very thick, almost paste-like cream that is essentially coconut milk with most of the water removed from it. It is made by chilling coconut milk and skimming off the thick, rich layer of cream that forms on top of it. It absolutely should not be substituted for coconut milk or coconut cream in recipes, although it could be substituted for condensed milk.

## HEART OF PALM

*Do hearts of palm come from coconut trees?*

They can. Heart of palm is a vegetable harvested from the inner core of a young palm tree. The tree is cut down, the bark removed, and the fiber around the tree's core is removed. What is left is a long, pale, cylindrical core: the heart of the palm. These are typically cut into smaller sizes and canned.

Because the tree is killed to get to the heart of palm, coconut trees are seldom used for their hearts anymore: They are more valuable when allowed to mature and grow coconuts. Domesticated peach palms—often grown on plantations in Costa Rica—are the most popular source of heart of palm today.

*What do people do with hearts of palm?*

This is a great question! The only thing I do with them is slice them into salads. Well, because they remind me of artichoke hearts, I put them on antipasti plates, too. Some people slice them into stir-fried dishes and curries.

## COCONUT COPRA

*What is copra? It sounds like a type of dance.*

It does, doesn't it? Copra is the dried meat, or kernel, of the coconut that is used to extract coconut oil. This isn't any old coconut meat; it's specially prepared coconut meat. Coconuts are split in half and drained of water, the shell removed, and the chunks of meat dried, typically on drying racks on the same plantation where they were grown, though sometimes the drying is done in kilns. From there, the coconut is pressed for oil.

## COCONUT CAKE

*I've heard that people feed cows something called coconut cake. Could farmers really feed cows cake?*

No, not really. Though they can—and do— feed cows and other livestock an extremely tough, fibrous food called "coconut cake" or "copra cake." It's not cake as we know it. Copra cake is a by-product of the coconut oil industry: Once the oil is extracted from copra, the remaining coconut cake is 18 to 25 percent protein, but it contains so much dietary fiber that it can't be comfortably digested by humans.

## COCONUT HUSKS

*Are coconut husks and coconut coir the same thing?*

Kind of. Coir is the name for the individual fibers that make up the shaggy husk.

The coir from young coconuts is wispier and white in color and is used to make body exfoliating brushes, formed packing material, and "bio-logs," which help control erosion.

*What does the word "coir" mean?*

The word "coir" comes from the Malayalam word *kayar* and the Tamil word *kayieu*, both meaning "rope" or "cord."

*Although I have no problem eating coconut products, when I touch coconuts, I get a rash. Is it possible to be allergic to the husk?*

Yes it is. The husk contains a natural form of latex, and some sensitive people may get a rash, redness, a bit of swelling, itchiness, or a combination of these when they touch it. If you have a contact allergy (or sensitivity) to latex, wear gloves when handling coconuts. Or make somebody else handle them for you!

*Are coconut husks used for anything?*

Why yes, they are! Lots of things! The husks of mature (brown) coconut are often transformed into charcoal. They are also made into floor mats, netting, starter pots for seedlings, and matting used to stuff mattresses and other furniture. The coir itself is popular for making scrub brushes and industrial floor and wall brushes.

## COCONUT SHELL

*What's the difference between a coconut husk and a coconut shell? Or are they the same thing?*

They are actually two different outer layers of the coconut. The husk is the outermost layer. It's the rough, shaggy covering you see on mature, brown coconuts. The shell is the smooth wood right under that.

*I have heard that every part of the coconut tree is usable. What are the shells used for?*

Many different things! They are carved into beads, buttons, and tiles for craft projects. They are often used as caves and other structures in home and commercial aquariums. In fact, octopi near the Indonesian coast have been seen using coconut half-shells as mobile homes. The creatures use tentacles to grasp and carry parts of the shell while traveling and then simply set up their "nut homes" when needed.

In countries that use and export a lot of coconut, the shells are made into a type of lightweight, long-burning charcoal brick, which is then used for cooking. Coconut shells can also be turned into activated charcoal, which has the unusual ability to absorb large amounts of impurities from gases and liquids. This is why it is often used to make filters for gas masks.

Coconut shells are also pulverized and added to other ingredients that are used to make plywood or fillers for plastics.

# COCONUT WOOD

*I keep hearing all of these wonderful things about bamboo wood for flooring, furniture, and home accessories. Can coconut palm wood be used in the same way?*

Yes. In fact, there is a growing market for coconut lumber or coco lumber (also known as cocowood). More and more builders, floor-covering companies, furniture makers, and designers of housewares are using coconut palm wood.

Coconut timber comes from farmed plantations of old coconut palms that no longer produce coconuts. In the past, millions of unproductive coconut palms (the palms usually reach this state at about seventy years of age) were felled each year and used as firewood or left to rot. Using them for building and home furnishings creates a new income source for plantation owners and is great for the environment.

*I have some beautiful coconut wood salad bowls. I'd like to use them, but don't know how to wash them.*

Care for coconut wood bowls, trays, platters, cutting boards, and utensils just as you would other wood items: No soaking, no dishwasher, no harsh soap, no abrasive scrub brushers or cleansing pads, no overly hot water. Dilute a pea-size amount of mild dish-washing soap in a few cups of tepid water. Apply with a sponge and rinse off. Towel-dry off excess moisture and allow bowls to fully dry before stacking. If, at any point, your bowls look stained, gently rub in a paste of kosher salt and water, and sponge off with a damp sponge. Should bowls look dry, massage a bit of coconut oil into the wood.

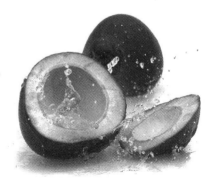

# COCONUT FOODS AND INGREDIENTS

http://www.artisanafoods.com/

Artisana sells yummy coconut butter and oil, as well as a range of interesting nut butters, such as walnut butter.

http://www.bobsredmill.com/

I get my coconut flour and dried coconut (flakes, shreds, and fine macaroon coconut) from Bob's Red Mill.

http://coconutbliss.com/

One of the most delicious lines of coconut ice cream around. Available in well-stocked grocers across North America.

https://www.coconutsecret.com/

The place for harder-to-find coconut ingredients, such as aminos, vinegar, sugar, and more. Also offers health and nutrition info, recipes, trivia, resources, and more.

http://www.edwardandsons.com/

Edward & Sons is the parent company for Native Forest, which offers the best coconut milk around and one of the only canned coconut creams on the market. Rich, made from organic coconuts, and free of the binders and fillers that cheap coconut milk has, this is my go-to brand. I love that the cans are BPA-free. Another of the company's brands is Let's Do . . . Organic, which features unsweetened coconut in various flakes, flour, and (in aseptic boxes) creamed coconut.

http://www.harmlessharvest.com/

My favorite coconut water. I love that it doesn't contain any sweeteners, chemicals, or other unwanted ingredients. Just organic, unheated coconut water.

http://navitasnaturals.com/

Navitas is "the" superfood company. Its coconut offerings include sugar and powdered coconut water—the only place I've seen the latter.

http://www.nikkiscoconutbutter.com/

Artisanal flavored coconut butter and nut-coconut combinations, all made in small batches.

http://www.kelapo.com/

High-quality organic extra-virgin coconut oil. Good stuff!

http://www.skinnycoconutoil.com/

Skinny coconut oil is high-quality, cold-pressed coconut oil made in small batches.

https://store.nutiva.com/

Nutiva sells all kinds of superfoods, from chia to goji berries, but we love the fun coconut products, such as Coconut Manna. Yum, yum, yum!

http://sodeliciousdairyfree.com/

SO Delicious offers a wide line of coconut milk in cartons and aseptic boxes, coconut kefir, coconut yogurt, and coconut ice cream. These products are available in markets across North America.

http://www.tropicaltraditions.com/

Tropical Traditions has a wide range of coconut oils and other coconut products (coconut tooth cleaner, anyone?) for cooking, the body, and the home. Books, too!

http://www.wildernessfamilynaturals.com/

A great online one-stop shopping spot for a wide range of coconut products.

http://www.earthcoco.com/

Sweeteners, raw coconut cream, raw coconut water, and one of the only places I've seen raw coconut meat, Earthcoco is a great resource for the coconut lover.

## COCONUT WISDOM WEBSITES

http://www.coconut.com/

This website, which bills itself as "the web guide to the tropical world" celebrates those places where coconut grows. But yes, there are also tons of coconut-based recipes.

http://coconutoil.com/

CoconutOil.com is a great source for current research and past studies on coconut oil and its effects on human health.

http://www.coconutresearchcenter.org/

The Coconut Research Center is dedicated to sharing ancient wisdom about coconut and its many traditional uses as a medicine and healing agent. There are also plenty of modern studies to read, recipes, crafts, trivia, and so much more.

http://www.kbakauai.org/

Kapaa, on the Hawaiian island of Kauai, is home of a coconut festival. Every October, people gather to celebrate coconut with food, education, crafts, entertainment, and more.

## COCONUT PREPARATION TOOLS

http://www.chefscatalog.com/

Chefs Catalog doesn't offer a lot of tools to help with coconut, but it is one of the only online suppliers in North America that carries the coconut knife.

http://www.youngcoconuts.com/

Not coconut-made products, but products that help you enjoy coconuts, including coconut scrapers, shredders, de-meaters, coconut noodle makers (I still am not sure what this is), and more.

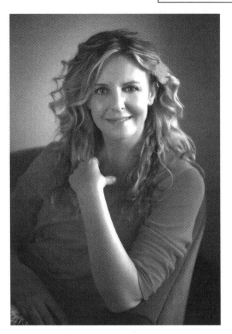

*Stephanie Pedersen, MS, CHHC, AADP,* is a holistic nutritionist, cookbook author, and corporate speaker. Author of more than twenty books, Stephanie has a reputation for giving her private and corporate clients the edge they need to get whatever they want from life. She does this by helping individuals lose weight, manage food allergies, and detoxify naturally, using food and lifestyle changes.

As Stephanie says, "I want health for everyone! I have seen firsthand with myself and my own clients that when one works to get clean and fit and address one's health challenges, life gets bigger. Suddenly, life becomes outrageously fun and easy. You move healthfully through life with ease."

According to Stephanie, getting healthy doesn't have to be complicated or time-consuming. "As a mother, writer, nutritionist, PTA mom, and someone who loves to have time alone to wander local farmers' markets, I know that complicated, overly fussy diets, or an unnatural obsession with calorie-counting, are not the answers to getting and staying healthy." Instead, Stephanie espouses a life of love, laughter, daily exercise, and your favorite whole foods. (Including plenty of coconut!)

"We're lucky that we live in a time when more and more gorgeous whole food ingredients, organic produce, and humanely farmed meat are available. Let's celebrate our good fortune by exploring our many food and fitness options and experimenting with abandon."

Pedersen currently lives in New York City with her husband and three sons. Visit her at www.StephaniePedersen.com.

## Also by Stephanie Pedersen:

*Kale: The Complete Guide to the World's Most Powerful Superfood*

*KISS Guide to Beauty: Keep It Simple Series*

*Ginseng: Energy Enhancer*

*Garlic: Safe and Effective Self-Care for Arthritis, High Blood Pressure, and Flu*

*Shoes: What Every Woman Should Know*

*Bra: A Thousand Years of Style, Support and Seduction*

## ACKNOWLEDGMENTS

I couldn't have finished *Coconut: The Complete Guide to the World's Most Versatile Superfood* without the support of my husband, Richard Joseph Demler, and our sons Leif Christian Pedersen, Anders Gyldenvalde Pedersen, and Axel SuneLund Pedersen. Thanks, too, to the NYC wellness community, which is a surprisingly tight-knit, happy group of healers who have reminded me to have fun as I have literally lived coconut for several months!

Thanks to my amazing clients for the constant inspiration you bring. Every day I am amazed at your drive, your courage, and your will. Getting healthy can be scary, and yet you see the joy in feeling your best, dive in, and create vibrant wellness for yourself. Yay, you! I am in awe of each of you.

I happen to have been working with a group of detoxers (hello 5-Day Detoxers!) during the last stretch of the *Coconut* manuscript, and the timing could not have been better: Coconut water coolers, coconut snacks, coconut oil–kissed veggies—all were springboards for fabulous detox conversations! I have never had so much fun doing a detox program or writing a book!

I can't say enough flattering (and true!) things about my gorgeous, good-humored, brilliant editor, Jennifer Williams. We go back in time through several publishing houses now. I count my blessings that I was assigned, as a young author, to you all those years ago. Here's to us! My designer, Philip Buchanan, ensured that the finished product was as polished and professional as possible. Bill Milne and Diane Vezza created the gorgeous mouthwatering food photos in *Coconut*. And my very thorough production editor, Kimberly Broderick, ensured the book you hold in your hands was as good as possible. Thank you! Your calm, can-do demeanors and overall smarty-pants ways make this crazy business of publishing look glamorous.

Thanks so much to my publicity pro, Sherri McLendon, of Professional Moneta. Sherri, I adore our monthly conversations. Not only are you fun and witty (and you know how much I love witty people), you make my professional life so much easier. Which in turn makes my professional life more fun!

Thanks, too, to every coconut grower and harvester—whether commercial farmer or weekend gatherer—who has ever lived. Without you, there would be no coconut chips. No coconut oil. No coconut water. No coconut milk smoothies. The world would be a less delicious place! Lastly, I must thank you, dear reader and coconut lover, for your interest. Thank you!

# INDEX

NOTE: Page numbers in *italics* indicate recipes.